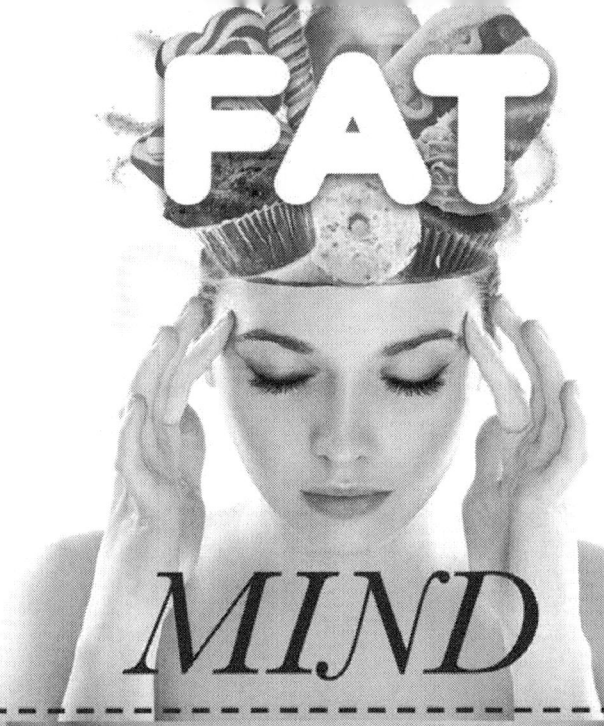

FAT MIND FAT BODY

International Bestselling Hypnotherapist,
Certified Nutritionist & Personal Trainer

BENJAMIN BONETTI

Benjamin Bonetti Ltd

First published in Great Britain 2012 By Benjamin P. Bonetti

www.benjaminbonetti.com

A catalogue of Benjamin Bonetti's work is fully available via all major online book suppliers

© Benjamin Bonetti Ltd 2012.

All rights reserved. No part of this publication may be reproduced, stored in a retrieval system, or transmitted, in any form or by any means, without the prior permission in writing of the publisher, nor be otherwise circulated in any form of binding or cover other than that which it is published and without a similar condition including this condition being imposed on the subsequent purchaser.

Every effort has been made to trace copyright owners. Please notify Benjamin Bonetti Ltd of any omissions and they will be rectified

dedicated to all those
trapped in a body they
want to change

Contents

Instructions	01
Chapter 1: NLP	09
What is NLP?	10
History of NLP	11
Why Diets Never Last	16
The Fundamental Effect	23
Why is Now the Right Time?	27
You Are Not Alone!	28
Modelling	29
Are You Towards or Away?	32
The Power of Language	36
Negative Language	37
Values and Believes	42
Setting Your Goal	43
Chapter 2: Nutrition	55
Introduction	56
Meal Size and Hunger Signals	60
Daily Nutritional Balance	64
Carbohydrates	67
Fats	75
Protein	84
Fibre	90
Five-a-day	94
Water	98
Chapter 3: Exercise	109

Why Exercise?	110
What Do You Enjoy?	114
Where?	118
When, How Long and How Often?	129
How Much?	123
Exercise Programmes	126
Old Wives Tales – True or False	148

Instructions

This book has been put together by a team of professionals to drive you forward, aiding you to produce massive results. By following the manual, step-by-step, it will take you on an educational journey to realign your values and beliefs and redesign the way that you look at your lifestyle and habits. The book has been designed for use in conjunction with the MP3s, where you will be asked to capture your thoughts and ideas as you progress and develop a better concept of your own mind. This simple system will help you maximise the benefits as well as your experience.

The book is written to reinforce specific ideas towards weight loss education and how they may be applied to your life, so if you were to browse through this programme now, it would make little or any sense to you. But when completed in a specific order, you'll find that each of the assignments will lead your thinking abilities on to an expanded level of personal progression. This book will not only help you achieve your personal weight loss goals, but will allow you to develop as a person, giving you skills that can be applied to all aspects of your life.

Be sure to take down any extra notes or ideas that may arise during your learning experience, so that you can refer back to them at a later date. You will find real value in putting your thoughts, ideas and emotions on paper. There is a certain amount of clarity that comes from writing something down no matter how silly, adventurous, or challenging it may seem. This is a highly simple yet rewarding system, proven to grow and expand your personal development. The more notes you write down, the more you will appreciate just how far you've come and the more you will become aware of your thoughts and feelings about the food you eat, what you eat, and why you eat.

"fat mind, fat body"

What is going to be involved, all depends on you as an individual, many things so often do. Different people have different requirements. Not everything within the book will be as relevant to you as other things. Some of the things are concepts you may do on a day-to-day basis but others may be new to you. It is going to be a collection of small changes that you're going to use to make an overall massive transformation. The book is going to teach you about how to set achievable goals, which will not only help you to lose the weight you want, but also help change your life so that it stays off, about nutrition, and how what you eat can affect you in both a good way and a bad way, and how to carry out appropriate exercises to aid your loss of weight. You are going to enjoy every step of the way by achieving the results that you desire; your personal goals and dreams will become a reality.

The first hurdle is found deep within you, although it may seem simple to understand, it is normally the thing that is missed out of more conventional weight loss programmes, we are in essence an intellectual creature. Within this programme, it is essential that you look to improve your overall wellbeing, not just your perception and image. How you feel on the inside is a direct reflection of your projection on the outside.

Before you start on your journey, you need to begin by being completely honest with yourself. With honesty and integrity you will be able to build a much better relationship with yourself and your body as well as equipping yourself to take action to change. Generally, people who lack personal integrity and honesty deny their own reality and lie to themselves, about their lives, their weight, and their psychological reliance on food. To change anything in your life, you need to confront your fears and denials, and never give in; this is the cornerstone of this programme. Remember for all intense purposes, there are never negative personal statements, just those that motivate you to do better and those that are fulfilling.

Instructions

You cannot begin a journey without first knowing where you are and where you want to go.

Q. Do you deserve joy and happiness in your life?

Q. Can you be honest with yourself?

Q. What do you need to admit to yourself to move forward in your life?

Q. How is being overweight positively affecting you?

Q. Are you happy with your weight and what others think about your weight?

Q. How does this make you feel?

Q. Why is now the right time to lose weight forever and massively change your lifestyle habits?

Q. Why are you committed now to change?

Once you are honest with the person you are, the sooner you can follow a life that is aligned with your beliefs and desires, allowing you to experience true happiness and satisfaction. A number of people are not truly honest with their state and will often go to a great extent to avoid the reality around them, psychologists may attribute this to a concept called cognitive dissonance, the truth is people do this by lying to themselves and often spending more time avoiding the task than if they were to complete it in the first place. Avoid letting this be your mentality, as this will have a negative impact upon your weight loss goals.

Lying, although a powerful negative word is one way to minimise the short-term pain. Lying to yourself to make a bad situation *"fat mind, fat body"* ─────────────────────

better than it is but in the long term it is still going to be there, and until you are honest with yourself and do something about it, it will only get worse. We lie to ourselves in many different ways, although each can be avoided through honesty and personal integrity. Lying about your weight or issues is simply delaying the pain and the action needed in the future. Put it this way, if you are gaining weight, it's going to be harder to lose the weight the more you have gained, therefore more effort and time will be required for you to achieve your goals. The sooner you stop lying to yourself, the faster you'll achieve the results, and the body you desire.

Q. What was the last lie you told yourself?

Q. How could you have been honest to yourself, to make a change?

Q. What lies have you been telling yourself about your weight?

Q. Why have you been doing this?

Q. Are you going to change it?

We often experience unhappiness in our lives because there is something happening externally that makes us feel uncomfortable, instead making excuses and leaving us to procrastinate. You must take action whenever faced with such an experience and when dealing with weight control issues, the same can be said. When working with yourself, it's essential that you find the initial root cause of the weight gain and deal with this. In doing so, you'll avoid the repeat and yoyo weight gain that is common to most weight loss plans. By addressing underlying causes, you will make permanent changes and achieve your goals all the faster. You may find the external environments within your life are effecting how you feel on the inside. If this is the case, you know exactly what areas you need to focus on and where change needs to be made.

Q. What has made you gain weight and why?

Q. When did you know that weight was an issue within your life?

Q. What do you remember happening specifically?

Q. When could you have started to make the changes necessary?

Q. At what point in the past did you decide that you had gone past the point of no return?

Fixing a short-term issue with a lie, leads to you failing to take appropriate action that could have remedied the situation. As you may have experienced in the past, this leads to the initial issue becoming a much bigger problem, in this case weight gain. Confronting your issues and problems straight away will give you solutions, as every problem has a solution, and a problem cannot arise without a solution. Your decision-making skills will become more acute, your character will strengthen and your confidence will grow until you achieve the perfect weight. The aim by the end of this programme is to ensure that you have highlighted the areas that need immediate attention, you have a basic understanding of nutrition and you are able to recognise that fitness isn't a chore but a positive life choice.

Remember, change is a positive thing and a natural part of everyone's life. We change each day, every time we meet someone new, every time we step outside the door. Change colours our lives and paints us with a full palette of experiences. Change is as natural a part of life as each breath we take, each inhalation and exhalation. Change is life.

Here are a few tips for getting the most from this book:

Resist jumping several pages ahead during the process. If your mind is thinking about the future, it's not focused on the present, and it is in the present where we make changes. Dealing with one thing at a time is all that is required.

Take a note of every thought you have, even if it doesn't make sense. Some of the most successful breakthroughs are started or developed with a thought. These thoughts may not make sense at the moment but will act as good reference points when you are successfully looking back in the future at how you changed and achieved your goals.

Write down any useful tips and how you can apply them in reality to your lifestyle. Remember we are all individuals and such tips are most useful when they can apply directly to our lives. These tips may include how you will overcome certain issues, perhaps include step-by-step notes of what you can do directly after completing the programme, and what you have learnt from that can be applied to other areas of your life as well.

Be specific with detail, the subconscious mind only works towards the specifics you give it. This includes dates, times, weights, locations, and people. The more specific you are, the more likely it is you will take real action and with real action there comes real change.

Hypnosis Instructions

Throughout this journey, we are going to ask you to listen to hypnosis to aid in your confidence and your weight loss process. Each of these processes has been specifically designed to assist you on your journey. Of course it is not necessary to listen to these, however those that have, have noticed a significant increase in their ability to keep the weight off for good, and remember it is through permanent change that we achieve success.

Within the Confidence Hypnosis recording, we will reprogram your mind to feel more comfortable and relaxed in social situations, believe in yourself, and achieve your full potential. You'll notice after just a few completed sessions that you will increase your belief that you deserve to walk with your head held high and have confidence in your stride. By listening to this hypnosis recording you can release your insecurities and experience a new way of thinking and feeling and achieve the weight you desire.

With our weight loss hypnosis recording, we reprogram your mind to achieve your goals, allowing you to easily turn down negative and harmful foods. You'll learn to see food as a valuable source of energy, not as something to turn to when you don't know what else to do, and you will achieve your sustainable target weight faster than if you had gone it alone. After just a few completed sessions with this audio, you'll start to pause before eating, your food portions will become smaller and you will feel fuller for longer. You will be taking that first and most important step towards permanent weight loss.

Tips for Listening to the MP3:

Pick a Time and a Place - Choose a safe place to listen to your MP3. Choose somewhere you can relax without being disturbed for 40-45 minutes. Many people like to listen to their MP3s before bedtime, others listen in the bath – but everyone is different.

Listen, Relax, Enjoy - Put on some headphones (highly recommended), lay back and listen to the hypnotherapy session.

"fat mind, fat body"

Just relax and let go, trying not to think consciously about what is being said as your unconscious (subconscious) mind will do all the positive work on your behalf. You may notice that it takes a couple of attempts to get into the swing of the patterns and the "not" thinking.

Repeated Listening - Each day for two weeks listen to the hypnosis MP3s which were downloaded with your pack to increase your confidence and help aid weight loss. Below is an outline of when to listen to each MP3, if however you notice that one audio has more effect than the other, you can change the process to suit you. Remember, this is a personalised programme.

Hypnosis Timetable:

Monday to Friday – Weight Loss Hypnosis

Saturday – Confidence Hypnosis

Sunday – Rest

So when you're ready to finally put poor eating behind you and take back control of your weight once and for all, relax, clear your mind of any preconceived ideas, and look forward to applying the skills you're about to learn.

Downloads: To download your hypnosis audio's, please register as a member on our website: **www.benjaminbonetti.com/members**

Once you have created an account, please fowward a copy of your purchase order to **info@benjaminbonetti.com**, with the subject title: **FATBODYFATMIND**. The downloads will be added to your account within 48hrs.

Chapter One

NLP & Lifestyle

What is NLP?

NLP stands for Neuro-Linguistic Programming, which encompasses the three most vital areas in producing the human experience. To utilise NLP within weight management, you must first understand its meanings, purposes and concepts. In brief:

Firstly, **Neurology**, which occurs within the brain. Within NLP we say that by increasing our awareness of the patterns in our thinking, we can learn how thought patterns influence the results we are getting in work and in life. The key therefore to finding personal health and success, comes primarily from within us.

Learning about "how" we think enables us to tap into our inner resources and find the results we truly desire. Using our thinking patterns in this sense, we are able to guide our awareness in the effective management of our weight and control the intake of food based on our thoughts alone.

The most effective tool in achieving your weight loss goals is the power of your mind.

Secondly, the **Linguistic** segment of NLP explains that our language is our life. What we can say is what we can think and what we can do. Learning to understand and master the structure of our language is essential in a world where we trade increasingly through our ability to communicate. Poor internal language, unfortunately, is a trait of those with weight issues, as explained later within this book, and is therefore something we must ensure is properly mastered.

Working to improve your language will provide you with the results you desire and improve your general outlook on life.

Finally, the **Programming** portion of NLP relates to the way we run our lives. We run our lives by strategies, similar to the way a computer uses a program to achieve a specific result. By understanding the strategies by which we run our lives, we gain the ability of choice – choice to do more of the same, or choice to take the necessary action to enhance our potential and our individual excellence; the choice to slowly increase our weight or the choice to increase our vitality, our fitness, our appearance.

Re-programming your internal strategies will define clarity and create perfect habits.

In essence, NLP is the study of our thinking, behaviour and language patterns so that we can build sets of strategies that work for us in making decisions, building relationships, starting up and developing goals, coaching a team of people, inspiring and motivating others and ourselves, creating a balance in our lives, negotiating our way through the day and, above all, learning how to learn change for the better.

By using NLP within weight management/control, you will achieve more of what you really want and become more of who you truly are. **Excellence is context specific.** Many diets fail because they assume that what works for one person will work for another, yet what makes a leading health plan successful for one person may be quite different to what constitutes success for another. NLP enables you to code excellence and enhance it, so that you can establish what really works for you in your environment and with your lifestyle.

History of NLP

So where did all of this come from? NLP became a collection of the works of John Grinder and Dr Richard Bandler, who studied

"fat mind, fat body"

the works of Virginia Satir, Fritz Perls, and Milton H Erickson, and packaged together a collection of processes that revolved around the development of behavioural competence and flexibility. Included in this were processes that allowed people to take on skills for the development of individual excellence; allowing the establishment of empowering beliefs, how communication works on many different levels, and what the process of change is all about.

After studying historic figures from many different fields, and collecting together a different theory, a package was produced, now known as NLP. Below are a few concepts that may enlighten you on your task ahead. The concepts have been incorporated within the writing of this book to ensure that you gain the most out of that which you wish to achieve.

"The map is not the territory."

The map is not the territory. This is a concept that explains: reality is never truly understood by any human, we only truly know our own perceptions of reality. Due to our sensory representational systems (what we hear, taste, see, smell, and feel), we respond to reality based on how we perceive it and therefore nobody's reality is the same. It is not reality itself that drives us or limits us, but the way that we distinguish reality. If the territory is reality itself then the map we draw is a map drawn by our sensory systems.

"There's no such thing as failure."

People within the world of NLP also like to spread the word that there is no such thing as failure, there is only feedback. On approaching a task, if you could only succeed at it, or learn for the next attempt, how many more things would you carry out in your life? If you approached a task and by the end, learnt a more efficient way of carrying it out next time, what would be stopping you from having a go at everything you have ever wanted to?

Q. What have you not done in your life because you were scared of failing?

Q. What more would you have done if you couldn't fail at anything?

Q. How much more successful would you have been?

NLP utilises trial and error, whereby not everything we do is going to work, though we explore the way in which we are going to make it work, and the results each time are a valuable source of learning. A prime example is Edison on inventing the light bulb. Trial, error and improvement not only lead him to his intended goal, but allowed him to create many more inventions along the way. The same can be said about your attempts to lose weight in the past; some aspects of alternative weight loss programmes may have been more effective for you than others. Combining your experiences and utilising the aspects that work for you is simply a trial and error process, it's not right or wrong, good or bad, positive or negative, simply a learning process on channelling the best system that suits your lifestyle.

"You already have all the tools you need to succeed."

The most influential theory of NLP for anyone who wants to succeed in life is that people already have all the resources they need to succeed, and in this sense, you already have all of the tools you need to lose weight. Once you believe this, then any change is possible, and to believe that you have all the resources you need is only dependent on your personal sensory representational systems. Anybody can change his or her reality if they believe, as the map is not the territory. Most of us just need to utilise what we already have in a different manner in order to achieve what we really want.

"fat mind, fat body"

If you think about a time when you needed to achieve something, your mental thinking immediately directed you to where you may find the answers. In this situation, you simply looked outside of the normal boundaries within your life and found the answers elsewhere. This will become more apparent the further you go within your weight loss programme; some things will put you outside your comfort zone, but this is fine, and remember the theory that you can't fail.

The ingredients and capabilities are within us, however, more often than not we need to change the steps we take or learn new ones. More specifically, NLP can support you in learning how to do the following:

• Accelerate your ability to learn so that you can not only manage change but also initiate and embrace it, enabling you to lead the way in your particular lifestyle.

• Continually develop new ways of thinking that support you whatever the changes in the external world.

• Let go of the old, traditional patterns and habits that constrict your growth and release the hidden talents that are appropriate to today and the future.

• Embrace feedback in a way that enables you to develop new ideas and habits with the involvement of friends and family.

• Set compelling outcomes for yourself; ones that by their very nature take on a momentum of their own and maximise the chances that you will achieve what you want.

• Develop formulae for yourself to enable you to respond to and more importantly, take a lead in the world of high technology, such that you combine the best of high-tech thinking with awareness of yourself and others.

• Build high-quality relationships with significant people in all contexts of your life, whether that be face-to-face or socialising in the 21st Century.

• Heighten your awareness of yourself and others, so that you are sensitive to the subtle shifts in behaviour and attitude that provide feedback on the effects of the way you communicate.

• Develop your flexibility so that you have more choices and consequently more influence over the situations in your life. Excellence is context specific.

• Improve your ability to generate commitment, co-operation and enthusiasm with yourself and the people around you.

• Manage your thoughts and feelings so that you are in control of your emotions and your destiny.

• Develop your ability to tap into your unconscious mind and draw on its superior power and potential.

• Accept and love whatever you have, and in so doing love yourself. Then you will be able to love others in a way that will transform your life.

Understanding why you do what you do is important during any learning experience, but as we all have different goals and objectives, not one weight loss plan alone can be designed to cater to the different specifics of each person. Therefore, within this programme, we have provided you with as much information and theory as possible, so you can adapt and personalise your journey. It may seem fairly content heavy, however, remember, the more information you hold, the more motivated you will be to achieve.

"fat mind, fat body"

Within weight loss, knowledge is power, the power to achieve your goals.

Knowledge is power.

It's well understood that by making clear statements about what you want to achieve, you realign your mind to pay attention. Just as you would notice a similar vehicle more often just after taking delivery of your own, throughout this book you will only take in the bits that are relevant to your future, some standing out more than others in the limitless journey of your mind.

Before you go any further, please make five content specific statements about what you aim to achieve during this programme, ensuring that you write each one in a positive context. Your mind will accept working towards something positive and will be more receptive to the change.

1._____

2._____

3._____

4._____

5._____

Why Diets Never Work

I am sure that no one who starts on a weight loss journey will ever want just a short-term result. They will actually want the weight they lose to stay off, and want to succeed in being a new, healthier person. Unfortunately, a diet alone isn't the answer to a permanent healthy lifestyle. If, for example, you eat healthily but you fail to exercise and you have a stressful life, then your diet isn't going to work. It's unlikely you'll stick to any weight loss plan unless you make a real change to your lifestyle; a real change to you.

Likewise, if you exercise but you eat a poor diet, then this also isn't going to work. It is essential that you combine a change that covers all three elements – diet, exercise, lifestyle – and works towards your overall goals, therefore leading to a healthier, better you.

Take my word for it, diets alone are only a short-term solution. Very few actually give you a long-term or lasting result, however tempting the latest fad diet may be. Promises of immediate results or rapid weight loss are hard to resist but if you ever consider dieting in the future, it's important to look more closely at the facts and long-term health aspects of any diet plan you choose to follow. You may well discover that the current fad diet could be causing you more harm than good.

There are many different approaches to weight loss on the market right now, all with their own unique formula to instant results such as the plethora of diet supplements, detox diets, low carbohydrate diets, low calorie diets, and group weight loss schemes, all of which can lead to you feeling that you have achieved your goals – but for how long?

The likelihood is that you will have tried at least six of these diets in the past, all with short-term results, and all creating a general sense of being let down, hence the tendency to continue jumping from one to the other. With this programme, (providing you have decided to change and know you want to change rather than know you should change), you will see permanent and lasting results. It may not happen as fast as with alternative methods but, overall, it offers lasting effects. Change is best when it is a permanent change for the better.

Q. Have you ever been on one of the diets listed above?

Q. Did it work for you?

Q. If so, for how long?

Q. If it didn't work, what could you have done differently?

Q. Which aspects of your previous diets did you enjoy?

Q. Which aspects of your previous diets did you find the most challenging?

It's worth noting at this stage that although diets involving meal supplements can be effective, especially if you are looking for a short-term fix or a kick-start, in the long run these diets fail to solve the real problems behind the initial weight gain, and therefore if possible should be avoided.

From experience, these diets fail to teach you good healthy eating habits or how to control the size of your meals, all key aspects of the reasoning behind real weight loss support. If, of course, they are supporting you as you look to divide the meals up into smaller regular meals (up to six per day) then they can work in favour of effective management of your metabolism. Let's face it, it isn't always convenient to have a healthy helping of food stashed away in your bag but a small shake can work just as well. However, if you use supplements as a main meal and then decide to come off the diet, it is very easy to slip back into your earlier bad habits and again increase your intake of larger portions. This is covered in more detail later within the portions section contained in the nutrition segment of the programme. If you are taking off-the-shelf supplements at the moment, please stop now.

Chapter One

Do I need to Detox?

A common topic of weight management that is always considered or discussed at least once within a weight loss résumé is the effectiveness of the Detox on our bodies, and do we have the need to Detox our bodies on a regular basis?

Overall, unless recommended by your doctor or physician, a Detox should be avoided. Detox diets are very good at stopping our body taking in certain food groups, but this can often lead to an inadequate intake of certain vitamins and minerals, all of which are essential to our body and are generally already lacking in a poor diet. Under normal circumstances, a healthy liver does all the "Detoxing" that is necessary for the human body. Although there is some justification to the suspension of unhealthy behaviours until your body starts to regain the level of nutrition that is needed to support the new you, a Detox diet is best avoided.

Do I need to cut out carbs?

Reducing your carbohydrate intake to aid in reducing your weight is seen as beneficial. This is because your body starts to find energy in alternative areas, conveniently using fat stores instead, although protein stores may also be used in extreme cases. However, the side effects may overpower your desire to lose the weight, with symptoms such as mood swings, tiredness, bad breath and headaches. On top of this, the rapid weight loss associated with cutting out carbohydrate is rarely sustained. In fact, low carbohydrate diets are notoriously difficult to sustain for more than a few months.

Imagine this scenario: you are eating out with a friend and all of a sudden the dreaded menu appears, the menu that you know contains no or very few appropriate meals for your diet – it's this feeling of dread, or fear, that makes relapse inevitable.

Low carbohydrate diets are also very often over-hyped. Evidence shows that such few carbohydrates are needed for the much-touted extra calorie burning effect due to protein's harder digestibility that the diet at this level is untenable. Some people may speak highly of this diet, and individuals do differ, but few people can lead the low carbohydrate lifestyle for long. In addition, by excluding many fruits and vegetables, there is a real risk that some low carbohydrate diets might result in vitamin and mineral deficiencies in the long run.

Do I need to count calories?

The low-calorie diet, like the Detox diet, excludes many food groups that are high in calories. Once again, this can lead to excluding many vital minerals and vitamins but more worryingly, it could lead to malnutrition if followed excessively. If too few calories are consumed each day, the body begins to conserve fat as a reserved energy source, and also begins to burn protein, such as muscle, when the calorie intake is below around a thousand less than needed for energy balance. After the diet, when food begins to be consumed on a normal level, weight is rapidly put back on. This is because the body needs to replenish depleted energy sources and, as it now fears for future starvation, fat levels are also restored in preparation for survival. Such diets can also be hard to follow, as by cutting calories alone without increasing requirements through exercise, you need to cut more to lose weight. This can be a large lifestyle change for someone to take, making it psychologically very challenging. When you then imagine a life of always having to count the calories, always having to check, always having to add, and always having to calculate, you find another reason why these diets often fail.

Chapter One

So the answer to the problem of dieting is that they are all unique and each have their own merits, finding their own way to help you lose weight, but, unless you are willing to carry out one of their schemes forever, then they may not be for you. The key to real weight loss is education and real lifestyle change involving both exercise and healthy eating, learning how to treat your body so that it can turn out exactly the way you want it in return.

Why This Programme is Going to Work For You, and You Can Say Goodbye to Diets Forever...

This programme is not only going to aid you through explaining what to do to lose weight, it's also going to educate you so that you feel completely confident in knowing how to keep the weight off for good. So far, we have proven that simply telling you the broad answers to effective weight loss isn't going to be enough.

You know that eating fatty foods isn't good; you also know that a lack of exercise isn't helpful, and finally, if your lifestyle isn't supportive to healthy living then it's not sustainable. However, this programme is about creating a better understanding of what works for you as an individual and overall establishes choices that you are going to have to make in order to achieve your weight loss goals and the perfect you. Today, we have more gyms, diets and resources that guide us towards healthy living than ever before, yet obesity is more of an issue than ever before. One contributing reason is choice and social acceptance.

If cutting out 80 per cent of your fatty food intake isn't a choice that you're prepared to take, then it doesn't matter what weight loss programme you choose, they are all likely to fail.

I am not telling you that the things you have tried in the past are wrong or don't work but that they will not give you the long-term results you aspire to: they lead to temporary change, not the permanent change you desire. Remember, as knowledge is power, the education gained from this programme will allow you to achieve the long lasting results you truly deserve – unless of course you don't feel that you deserve to be fit, healthy, attractive and sexy. Your motivation for weight loss is an important guide to aid your focus on the journey you are about to undertake.

Q. What would you give to be emotionally free of weight?

Q. What are your motivators to losing weight for good?

Q. What will happen this time if you do not see it through?

Q. Who do you blame when things don't go the way you want?

Q. What would it feel like to complete this programme and keep the weight off?

So, the real question is; why, apart from emotional issues, do so many people have difficulty keeping the weight off?

The answer can be explained in simple terms; weight gain is a result of people eating or drinking more calories than they are using up during a day, in other words, they are in excess of their energy balance. If people consume large quantities of food or drink and the calories are not used up in the body's general maintenance and exercise carried out during the day, then the outcome is that the calories consumed are stored in the body, mainly as fat. Simple, isn't it?

More calories consumed than burnt each day = weight gain.

Think about it; if we eat more than we work off, then we will gain weight. However, for someone who has lacked physical exercise, the body has cleverly adapted to turn all food sources into fat as this is the body's preferred energy store. Our bodies' only need a certain number of calories to maintain us, this is called the basal metabolic rate. Energy balance is then calculated by multiplying the basal metabolic rate by a number representing our level of physical activity. The main aim of an effective weight loss plan is therefore to re-educate the body and kick-start the metabolism, ensuring that the right amount of energy is used compared to the amount of food consumed.

The Fundamental Effect

Pain is the most common reason why a person ends up wanting to take action on a problem, but not just any pain, when the pain hurts too much. Remember that pain can be either physical or mental. Each of us seems to have a different and an enigmatic capacity for pain. Some of us will die before changing and yet some of us change what we are doing the second we are slightly uncomfortable.

When this moment of "enough" occurs in our life, it leads us to actually act on the pain and do something about it. To act against weight issues, pain may be as simple as realising that your favourite pair of trousers no longer fit, that you are no longer able to keep up with your children in the park, or the extreme of generally feeling that your weight is preventing you from doing anything constructive with your life. You will therefore act on this pain as it has become too much, or maybe you are part of the unique few who want to avoid pain before it actually occurs and are taking action to prevent any problems in the future. Whatever your motivation for weight loss, it is this pain that provides the initial push many of us need.

"fat mind, fat body"

People may believe that they must do something about their pain but feel that they can't, often because of past failures, not knowing where to start, or having lost weight before only to have it come back on. When this is the case, it can lead to you telling yourself that you can't do something so many times that you actually start to believe it, and "can't do" effectively becomes a negative incantation. The truth is, you can do it, you are just trying to convince yourself otherwise.

Why is it So Hard For Many?

Many people I am sure have tried a variation of diets that may have worked for a period of time with reasonable results, but how long did the results last? Did you end up putting the weight back on? Even worse, did your diet produce no change in your weight at all? Why is this?

This may be because to improve, we must continuously change, and it must be a long-term achievement that is incessant. For this reason, rather than giving you something that will help you change for the meantime, this programme will change your life.

If you have not changed, it may also be because it is in our nature to resist change. People often find themselves looking for excuses, or employing the common reasoning of "waiting and seeing" as maybe something will change without taking action – has this ever really happened?

It is known that people are resistant to change as change takes them outside their comfort zone. The more they change, the further out of their comfort zone they become, therefore the more resistance they have to change. The greater the resistance, the more difficult it is to improve. Do you procrastinate and put off taking any action? Or perhaps tell yourself that you have a "weight condition," or lead yourself into believing that "just one more" won't harm you?

Q. What excuses do you give yourself on a daily basis that reaffirm you are fat?

Q. What does your weight restrict or prevent you from doing during the day?

We both know that change is what you desire and therefore it is essential to break the routine, the habits and the old lifestyle. If you are labelling what you are going to learn and achieve as a "diet" then it is only a matter of time until the old weight comes back on, and unfortunately it might bring along even more weight to add to it; but when you start to question your beliefs about food and adopt a more in-depth nutritionally focused approach towards the food you eat, you begin to pick up and understand the benefits, which in turn begins the process of changing your old, negative and limiting beliefs into positive, enlightening ones.

Linguistics is one of the most important aspects in training your mind to achieve the results you desire. What you label something can have a dramatic effect on how you perceive it. So to label something a diet, automatically tells your brain that there is a start and a finish, it is not a long-term fix but a short-term solution.

The word diet signifies only a temporary time in your life as every time you carry out a diet, there is a beginning and an end, and then you return to those old habits. You always give yourself a time limit of "I'm going to go on a diet for Lent," or "My new year's resolution is..." or "I'm going to lose 12 pounds" etc., and then the second you achieve it, you tell yourself, "Wow, that was easy, or hard, quick, slow, fun, or boring, and now I can go back to eating and drinking like I used to," irrespective of how bad your eating and drinking habits may have been.

You will also find that you have used some of the following statements within your past weight loss attempts.

- It's within my genes, everyone within my family is fat!

- My metabolism is slow. (This is not actually a medical fact, you're just guessing!)

- I can't exercise because I have asthma, weak joints, injury from when I was younger etc.!

- I can't shift the weight; I have tried everything!

If you dissect the language you use, including the statements above, you'll notice how these patterns of language are actually producing a self-evolving prophecy. The more you think about a statement being true, the more you will notice the events that confirm it. I am not saying that none of this is true – some people do have genetic differences, and some people do actually have slow metabolisms, however, taking the mass, only a very few would be medically diagnosed. If you are honest with yourself, it's most likely that you are not one of them.

No matter what your genetics, background, or budget, weight loss is achievable and you can obtain the results you desire.

I can't stress enough that a diet is only a temporary fix and therefore doesn't work. When you are committed to changing both your dietary and fitness lifestyle, you are preparing and adapting yourself for the long-term and in doing so are committing to changing your language. If you do make these changes it's a guaranteed weight loss formula. Think thin and you'll become thin, think fat and the inevitable will happen.

Q. What are you going to name the process you are about to take part in?

Q. Why do you really want to lose weight?

Q. How is losing weight going to change your life?

Why is Now the Right Time?

> *"The best time to plant a tree is 20 years ago. The second best time is now."*
> Chinese proverb

The wisdom of the above proverb can be applied to so many different segments of our lives, both personal and professional. If you had planted a tree 20 years ago, you could now be enjoying its shade and eating the fruits, but what if you didn't plant it 20 years ago? Surely now would be the best time?

Many people have plans of starting diets or intentions to go to the gym but never really get through to taking action. The question is why?

Will there ever be the perfect time to start something? How about right now, as there is no better time than now? Perhaps you have a priority list whereby starting your journey to your desired weight isn't as high as watching your daily TV programme. Perhaps you need to sit down and re-establish your priorities. Over the coming weeks, notice how much time you are committed to doing nothing and think about ways that you can do something, either educational or physical. There probably is no better time to change your lifestyle, and the way that your life journey is going, than right now.

Q. Is there ever a perfect time to do something?

"fat mind, fat body"

Q. What is the difference between starting something new now, and putting it off until a later date?

Q. What are the excuses you have previously allowed to run your life?

Q. If you did not procrastinate, what would you like to start getting done right this moment?

Life does not care where you are or what you're doing; every now and again it will throw you a hand you just have to deal with. Like all of us, it's hard to start but once you start down the "positive" path, life gets easier.

If you always do what you always did, you always get what you always got.

Remember, your mind works towards the pleasures and away from the pain, but as you associated pleasure with poor nutrition and pain with physical exercise; the transition will inevitably cause some turbulence.

You Are Not Alone!

We can start by changing the way we think and feel about our body and ourselves. The Law of Attraction says that all our thoughts, all of the images in our mind, and all the feelings connected to our thoughts will later manifest as our reality. In other words; everything you have in your life☐now☐has been attracted to you through your mind, and everything you intend to achieve must also begin by you believing in yourself and attracting it.

We need to attract things into our life that we desire. We can do this by focusing on what we wish to create. If we focus on something that is undesirable, then we are more likely to attract that undesirable something and things that are unwanted into our life as we bring in the things we attract, both positive and negative, through focus. So, an initial step is to focus on what it is that you desire to achieve, making it possible to start making steps towards that vision. Realising that going to the gym and getting the body you want is possible, and easy, will start to make your body and mind work in partnership to achieve this, whereas believing the opposite will leave you in a position you don't want to be in. Negative thoughts beget negative consequences.

Modelling

If someone can do it, anyone can do it. That is the basis of modelling. Modelling is concerned more with the how than with the why. There is a joke that NLPers don't introduce themselves by saying, "How do you do?" but with, "How do you do that?" Modelling is a state of curiosity and selflessness. It is a desire to listen, watch, respect and learn from others as well as ourselves. Modelling is an interest in process over content.

Modelling is one of the most important skills we need in personal development.

More than ever before, we need to be self-reliant in the way we learn, develop, manage ourselves, take initiatives and cope with constant change. Even though you may have a close family, the chances are that no matter how much support you receive, you either already are, or most certainly will be, expected to be self-reliant in the way you respond to the challenges you face. There are few easy options in life and the pace is such that others are busy looking after themselves.

However, the good news is that most people have barely scratched the surface when it comes to drawing on their inner resources and few really know how to do this. Modelling is the answer. It is not just a technique, it is a lifestyle, such that wherever you are and whomever you are with, you can be learning and growing.

Modelling is a way of achieving lifelong learning and true personal fulfilment. It is a way of respecting the unique talents that we all have. There are powerful implications in the yardsticks we use to "box" people into what is acceptable and what is not. Modelling goes way beyond a new test. It respects the fact that whatever talents we have are of value and can be directed toward our own good and for the good of others. To learn to model is to change the myths of IQ stereotypes. It is to learn to respect and allow everyone his or her rightful place in the world.

Modelling can take many forms. Modelling others will have taught you some of your most fundamental skills. Babies and young children are expert modellers. Only when they start learning by more traditional methods do they begin to lose this skill. You can model anything. People are excellent in many different spheres and can display numerous traits we desire for ourselves.

You can, for example, have excellence in the ability to:

• Generate commitment and respect.

• Motivate yourself and others.

• Sell and influence.

• Speak a language fluently.

• Communicate using the latest technology.

- Lead and inspire.

Equally, you can have excellence in your ability to:

- Get depressed.

- Sulk.

- Lose your temper.

- Remain untouched by emotion.

- Procrastinate.

- Resist change.

- Respond aggressively to others.

Q. Knowing this now, who is already achieving what you want?

By modelling any of the above, you can develop a conscious awareness of the process and with conscious awareness you have a choice: to continue the same process or to do something else. Merely the process of studying what we are doing and how we are doing it lifts us to a level of detachment in which we can choose what we do and more importantly, what we continue to do in the future.

Q. Knowing people you could possibly model, what aspects would you mirror in your own life?

We achieve the results we do through the programs we run in our minds and in our actions. Just as computer programs are a sequence of codes, so personal programs are a sequence of mental and behavioural codes. When you walk, talk, drive, read, or laugh, it is unlikely that you think consciously about how you do these things. The programs that make them happen are managed on your behalf by your unconscious mind. These programs are known as strategies.

If someone else can do it, then so can you.

Why can't you model yourself with somebody who has achieved what you must do or reached where you want to be? The answer is you can. But you need to ensure that the person you model is someone of excellence, and someone who has been through what you have been through.

There is no point in modelling somebody who has not been through the stages that you aspire to accomplish, you need to find someone who has made a successful transition.

Are You Towards or Away?

You are probably thinking, "what does this mean?" People can be placed into two different categories; they can either be a "towards" or an "away from" person, and can switch between the two but never be both at the same time. If you are a towards type of person, then you strive to achieve something that you want or desire, whereas if you are an away from person, your main aim is to work away from something that you don't want. There isn't one way that is better than the other, merely two different ways of looking at what type of person you are.

The most obvious example, in terms of helping you to clarify what type of person you are, is to establish the reason why you wake up every morning and go to work for a whole day to earn money. Is it to get away from bills and the financial commitments that your life has, or is it because you strive towards saving enough money to move into the bigger house you dream of, or new car you have been waiting to buy?

More specifically, are you changing your lifestyle and educating your mind to be healthy because you must get away from that feeling of pain and dissatisfaction when you try on certain clothes you no longer fit into; trying to get away from the uncomfortable feeling you have after finishing a meal you know wasn't good for you, even though it felt like such a good idea at the time? Or, are you working towards being able to complete the charity marathon that you have always wanted to do; getting back into an old dress you used to love, that you know you can get back into? Knowing whether you are a towards or an away from person can help you set out your goals more efficiently, as you realise what needs to be included in order to aid your success and achieve the results you desire.

The most successful people in weight loss are towards people, as this allows an individual to concentrate on working towards the positive and avoid thinking about the negative. Although neither an away nor a towards person is any better than the other, wouldn't it be nice to feel more positive? As mentioned earlier, you can be both, but not at the same time, so now is a good time to think about how you want to think about your future, and how you will focus yourself to achieve your results.

Currently, you may be a towards person, but the desire you work towards may be aligned towards the wrong thing. You may be working towards food, or if you are an away from person, you may be working away from health and exercise. With this understanding, goal setting will help you realign your ideas to the achievable results you want and deserve.

Q. Now knowing this, do you consider yourself a towards or an away from person?

"fat mind, fat body" ─────────────────────

Q. What are you working towards or away from in alignment with your health?

Q. What would be beneficial for you to work towards or away form to become the person you want to be?

Below you'll find a table with the layout of four different sections. As you have now established what type of person you are, be it towards or away from, you can now begin to fill this out by listing your present situation first. This means listing 10 things that you currently work towards, or 10 things that you currently work away from. They can be anything at all.

Then, once you have filled out the top half, fill out the bottom half by listing the things that you want to be. You may currently be an away from person but, on finishing this book, you want to be a toward person, so fill out this section by listing all the things you wish to work towards.

Present – Are you away from or towards? Fill the side that best suits you.

Towards (list 10)

_____

_____

_____

_____

Away From (list 10)

Chapter One

_____

_____

_____

_____

Future – Do you want to be away from or towards? Fill out the side that you would most like to be.

Towards (list 10)

_____

_____

_____

_____

Away From (list 10)

_____

_____

_____

_____

Q. Can you change the way you think?

Q. Is it okay to give yourself permission to change and take action?

Here's a real-life example:

Let's say you have a tough day at work, the boss disagreed with your new ideas for the company, you got stuck in traffic on the way home and you walk through the front door and relax on the couch. The first thing to recognise is that you are having uninspiring or negative thoughts about things you can't change. You need to realise that as quickly as you have these negative thoughts, you can replace them with more cheerful and positive thoughts.

Everybody has a choice on how they react in different situations and how you decide to act is up to you. People rarely think about the nature of their thoughts, yet the quality of what you think about determines the quality of the life that you live.

The Power of Language

Most people talk to themselves, not always out loud, but definitely inside their own head. These conversations with yourself are known as inner dialogue. By changing the way we talk to ourselves, we can massively change the way our actions are carried out. Saying things to yourself differently can change how you feel, how successful you are, and how likely you are to achieve your goals. You need to believe that change is a "must" and not a "should". Someone who should change is doing it because it is a convenience to them and they won't give it 100 per cent. But, someone who establishes that they must change also establishes the belief that they can change. If you don't believe you can do it, you won't put in anywhere near enough effort to complete your goals and get the body you desire.

Chapter One

Negative Language

The way we think about ourselves defines our self-esteem, so the way you think of yourself defines the feeling of pride you have in yourself, and the way you decide to communicate with yourself internally can directly affect whether you boost or lower your self-esteem. It all depends on the words you decide to use. Being able to give ourselves self-confidence is an easy thing to do, but even easier not to. Many people negatively communicate with themselves without even realising it, and to some extent it becomes a habit. This will in turn drag them down and prevent them from performing at their optimum.

Ideas, thoughts, or the way that you communicate with yourself internally are merely a question and answer process within the mind. If you control the questions you ask, then you also control the answers you give.

Q. Why can't I lose weight?

A. Because I am lazy!

Q. How can I lose weight and enjoy the process?

A. I can go to the gym, eat healthier foods, and meet like-minded people!

Words...

The words that you use must be empowering. Know what negative words are, and how they change the outcome of your internal communication. Negative emotions require more detailed thinking,

"fat mind, fat body"

more subtle distinctions.

We conjure up more negative words because the language we use needs to be precise, and research suggests this is probably true for every culture and every age group throughout the world. Even though some of these words may not have precisely the same meaning in every language, they still tend to be more negative than positive.

Write down, or circle below, 10 words or phrases that you use on a daily basis that would be classified as negative. Some examples include:

Ashamed, Beaten down, Cut down, Can't, Tried, Try, Cannot, Criticized, Dehumanized, Disrespected, Embarrassed, Humiliated, Inferior, Insulted, Invalidated, Labelled, Lectured to, Mocked, Offended, Put down, Resentful, Ridiculed, Stereotyped, Teased, Underestimated, Worthless, Bossed around, Controlled, Imprisoned, Inhibited, Forced, Manipulated, Obligated, Over-controlled, Over-ruled, Powerless, Pressured, Restricted, Suffocated, Trapped, Abandoned, Alone, Brushed off, Confused, Disapproved of, Discouraged, Ignored, Insignificant, Invisible, Left out, Lonely, Misunderstood, Neglected, Rejected, Uncared about, Unheard, Unknown, Unimportant, Uninformed, Unloved, Unsupported, Unwanted, Accused, Cheated, Falsely accused, Guilt-tripped, Interrogated, Judged, Lied about, Lied to, Misled, Punished, Robbed, Abused, Afraid, Attacked, Defensive, Frightened, Insecure, Intimidated, Over-protected, Scared, Terrified, Threatened, Under-protected, Unsafe, Violated, Cynical, Guarded, Sceptical, Suspicious, Un-trusted, Untrusting, Low.

What empowering/motivational words can you use to replace these?

Chapter One

Q. What are the most common negative words you use to describe yourself?

Q. Are these words true?

Q. Who are you really?

Q. Is this fair?

Q. Do you deserve this?

There are many examples of how we can communicate with ourselves in a positive way, and boost our self-esteem, such as just reminding ourselves of the things we are good at: I am successful, I am confident, or things that we will do, such as: I am able to succeed in completing this task, or I have the ability to finish this objective, or, most importantly, convincing ourselves of something we don't initially think we can do or may not find too interesting to carry out: This task is going to be difficult but I am going to enjoy doing it as it is a challenge and I love challenges.

If we continually talk to ourselves positively then it is near impossible for us to have a low self-esteem as we are always reinforcing the idea that all of our values are amazing, that we are uniquely positive people, and that every concept we hold is a benefit to our lives.

The problems arise when you start to doubt yourself or put yourself down: I can't do this, that won't work, or I shouldn't attempt it.

"fat mind, fat body"

These forms of communication will leave you almost definitely feeling worse, and every time you talk to yourself in this way, you are only going to lower your self-esteem and reduce your chances of being the successful, positive person you want to be. The worse part of conversing with yourself in this way is that the majority of the negative language you use towards yourself is false.

Think of a time when you have used the word can't or shouldn't. Every time you use the word can't in a sentence, you are actually telling yourself that you can do it, but you are just deciding not to. There is also nothing in the world that you want to do that you shouldn't do, what you are actually saying is that you should do it, but you're not going to for whatever reason you have decided to convince yourself of. The sooner you start reframing your life around avoiding this negative language, the sooner you will see massive changes in your self-esteem, behaviour and most importantly, results.

The ability to reframe a situation is being able to see the other side. This can be done in almost every situation you might face. There are often situations in our day-to-day lives when something may not go exactly to plan, but you can learn to reframe these situations to see the positive side.

State three questions you normally ask yourself, then reframe them to provide a different answer.

For example, "Why can't I lose weight?" reframed to "How can I lose weight and enjoy the process?"

1._____

2._____

3._____

Chapter One

So, what needs to be done? Initially, you need to start recognising when in your life you are second judging yourself, or preventing yourself from achieving truly great things. You'll probably find that one of the causes will be your internal communication. To build self-esteem, you need to change the way you talk to yourself.

Whenever you recognise yourself using negative language, rephrase the sentence in your head, then say it again and see how different you feel once it has been stated in a more positive tone.

A pet hate of mine that often comes up in life is the word "try". It is just an idea, and you may disagree, but it has been recognised over time that it is very rare for people who "try" to accomplish or achieve something, to come out with the results they truly desire.

The second that you try, you are opening your mind up to the possibility that you may fail. If you approach a task with a more positive attitude and remove the word try, then the chances of success are far greater as you are not allowing your mind to recognise that the potential for failure is there.

For example:

I am going to try to lose 12 pounds by Christmas this year.

By simply removing the word try, this becomes:

I am going to lose 12 pounds by Christmas this year.

Or, the statement becomes even more efficient by adding the word must:

I must lose 12 pounds by Christmas this year.

By changing your language to be more positive, it will give your brain a more secure goal to reach; a goal that will seem far more achievable. This will undoubtedly give you fantastic results, over and over again, true?

Q. How is changing your language going to assist you in carrying out your programme?

Values and Beliefs

Values are the creed on which a person's life is founded, and they are made up of a collection of the beliefs and ideals that have been established from the person's culture, upbringing and family, along with their own life experiences. Stealing may be unacceptable normally, but with no money, and hungry children to feed, one might steal for food and remain true to one's values.

Beliefs are a person's personal views about what they think is true and false for both the world and themselves. They are conceived ideas from their experiences that are then modified by their perceptual filters (generalising, distorting and deleting) giving them a finished product of what they suppose.

The difference between beliefs and values is that beliefs are what your values are based on. For example, your value might be food, as eating is essential to your survival, but your belief might be that you are going to eat healthy food, as it is better for you.

Thus what you believe determines what you deem valuable, whether it is human life, health, personal freedom, freedom of speech, or even money.

You need to determine that you have positive beliefs about yourself, as many of the limitations and successes you face in your life are

Chapter One

self-imposed by your beliefs. What you believe about yourself can either hold you back from accomplishing your goals, or drive you forward to succeed anything you wish for, anything you desire.

Right now you are probably thinking that you already have lots of positive beliefs and fantastic values that you have built up over the years of your life, but still you are not achieving the results you want. So, therefore, you need to ask yourself; what are my values and how have I prioritised each and every one of these values?

If there is a goal you wish to achieve, and the value in your life for what you would gain by achieving that goal is of minimal priority, then maybe you need to rethink and realign your priorities?

Setting Your Goals

Firstly, we need to specify exactly what we want to achieve so that it is crystal clear. We can sum this up by the five Ws (Who, What, When, Where, and Why). Although it seems silly to determine "who" because as you are reading this, it is quite clear that you are the one wanting to carry it out. When we are setting goals for ourselves the who is you!

We now need to actually create the goal, determining what we desire our end result to be. Whilst creating the goal, what we don't want to see is a generalised accomplishment; "I want to become fitter, stronger, and slimmer." The goal has to be specific so that your brain knows exactly what it is aiming for. "I want to be able to run five kilometres in 22 minutes by the XXth of March 20XX."

The more specific the goal, the more focused your mind will be towards achieving it.

Have you ever planned to do something over the weekend such as,

"fat mind, fat body"

"I must hoover the car," but then completely forgot to do it or put it off? The likelihood is, if you had planned a specific time to do it and a solid reason why it needed to be done, then you would have ensured that the weekend task was carried out, you would have achieved your goal.

Q. Specifically, what do you desire your end goal to be?

But why do you want to carry out this goal? This is the next question you need to ask yourself, as you need to find out the reason, the purpose, and the benefits behind carrying out the goal. If you have no real reason for doing it then your mind won't give it 100 per cent and you will be doomed to failure. Having a reason will drive you through the hard times and keep you on track to achieving your fitness goals. The more honest and meaningful the reasons why you want to achieve your goal, the more they will help you through any difficult periods when you may be considering giving up.

Q. Why do I want to reach my goal?

The desired end result has to be evaluated and any necessary additional changes need to be made to ensure that it is achievable, as the last thing we want is for all the hard work to be put in and your ultimate goal to be impossible to reach. This would only lead to de-motivation and failure. When setting our goal, we must be realistic. What we want to achieve has to be within our grasp because at the end of the day, we all want results. Yet on saying this, nothing is impossible, so what we need to do is ensure a balance between what we wish to achieve and how long we are giving ourselves to achieve it.

To help this process further, high achievers tend to set their goals differently. Rather than set goals that are very difficult to achieve, i.e. things that relate more to perfection than reality, they set goals that are possible. For example, rather than set a goal such as, "I must exercise every day," they set something like, "I must exercise three out of seven days a week." Another example might be, "I must stick rigidly to my meal plan" versus, "I can eat healthily based upon my meal plan at least five days in the week."

This is important because of the concept "success breeds success" and because you are constantly making comparisons between what you set out to achieve and what you actually achieve. If, when you look at the past, you have been successful, it helps you feel positive and good about yourself. On the other hand, if you haven't been successful, you may feel guilty and become discouraged. So often when you feel negative, it relates back to the expectations you set yourself.

Once you learn to get off your own back, paradoxically you will begin to achieve more.

Knowing this, you need to have a start date. You need to establish the exact time and date of when you intend to start reaching this goal. Having an exact start time will mean you can have everything planned out and in place for setting off towards your desired outcome. But, when setting that goal, ensure that you have finished this programme first, as that will ensure you have all the tools you need to achieve what you deserve. You will have learnt all the key points to help you change your lifestyle and avoid all of those bad habits. Then, once you have decided that key time to start, all you need to do is simply write it down. For example, "I will start this on the XXth September 20XX at 8.00am."

Q. When are you going to start your journey towards achieving your goal?

To commit yourself completely, you need to be able to picture in your brain, every aspect of the path towards accomplishing your goal, and this includes where you are going to do it. It is going to be

"fat mind, fat body"

a long-term plan, therefore it may be occurring in many different locations, so you must know where you need to be in order to achieve the goals you wish to achieve. Knowing where you need to be will keep you on task. Are you going to complete all of your exercises in the local park, on the beach, in the gym?

Have every aspect covered so there are no excuses; what happens if it rains, do you have a backup plan? What happens when the gym is closed? Remember there are many exercises you can do in your own home.

Also consider the places you wish to avoid, for example, fast food restaurants or places where you know you may fall back into your old lifestyle, like a bar or pub. It is important to have strategies for just such occasions.

Q. Where are you going to carry out your exercise programme?

Q. What is your plan B?

How are you going to know when the goal has been achieved? To be measurable, a goal must be written down. Not only so you know what you are achieving and when you are achieving it, but also so you have something to be proud of. Being fitter, stronger, slimmer is all very well, but without being able to know how much fitter, stronger, slimmer you wish to be and without a uniform way of measuring it, you will never know when you have achieved anything. Are you going to keep a record of your weight, take monthly photos of yourself so you can physically see the change, try on a pair of tight jeans that are currently a tight fit and see them getting looser and looser, or maybe carry out body fat tests?

Q. How will you know when you have achieved your goal?

Q. How are you going to measure this?

Not all of these tests are constructive, so be aware. There are some things that can increase your weight, causing it to fluctuate significantly from day to day, and this will obviously have an effect on your results:

• The body is about 60 per cent water and fluctuations in your hydration levels can change the number on the scale and even body fat percentage measured through electrical impedance. Also, if you're dehydrated or have eaten too much salt, your body may actually retain water, which can cause your body weight to creep up. Similarly, many women retain water during menstrual cycles, which can induce the scales to weigh you in at more than your true weight. *Some advice: standing on the scales with one foot doesn't seem to help either!*

• Weighing yourself after a meal isn't the best idea simply because food that you've eaten adds weight. It doesn't mean you've gained weight, it simply means that you've added something to your body, like standing on the scales whilst carrying your daily food shop in plastic bags. But don't worry; this will go down after a few hours of the digestion process-taking place. The best time to weigh yourself is in the early morning after a bowel movement and before breakfast, at the same time each week, skipping measurements during the menstrual period.

• Muscle is denser than fat and it takes up less space, so if on starting your newly changed life, you have started using the gym, adding muscle could increase your scale weight, even though you're slimming down, so keep this in mind as it is a common misunderstanding. Body fat is more accurately measured by skin fold callipers than bio-impedance scales and may be a more constructive way of keeping track of your fat weight.

Once your goal is written down, you must ensure that all of the

"fat mind, fat body"

words within your specific goal drive you towards achieving it. For example, "I shall no longer say I want to achieve, or I intend to achieve, but I *must* achieve." This will change the way in which you look at your goal and instead of it being something that has to be done along with all the other things you have to do within our hectic 21st Century lifestyle, your brain will prioritise it as something of high importance.

And, you must ensure that you do write your goal down. Once your goal has been established and you are pleased with it, it needs to be written down, as it is a fact that 95 to 97 per cent of people who set goals do not write them down and therefore are never going to achieve them, whereas the three to five per cent who do write down their goals, obtain the results they desire.

Now think of a place in your life that you look at on a regular basis and place your written goal there so you see it on regularly, reminding yourself of the goal you must achieve. This could be on your fridge, to make you think twice when deciding on what to snack on, or on your desk to remind you to go to the gym in your lunch break. Whichever works for you, but these simple steps will help carry you through to your desired result.

Q. *Where will you place your goal?*

Finally, all you have to do is tell people; let people know what you are setting out to achieve, and be proud of it, as this will drive you to achieve it. Adding this accountability will often be a motivator in itself, because naturally, as humans, we don't like to fail, especially when people are counting on us. Where you can, add as much positive pressure to your achievement as possible, perhaps lose weight for charity or work towards taking part in a physical event such as a fun run or marathon.

Remember it takes small steps to cross the pond...

Chapter One

Establishing a long-term goal is a huge step forwards but to make it easier to achieve, we can now break it down into smaller chunks or stepping-stones, so you have a collection of short-term goals to reach success. There is no point trying to leap over a large pond and getting your feet wet. Isn't it far more practical to have a clear path for your mind to follow, keeping yourself nice and dry? Keep this analogy within your mind and whenever faced with a challenge repeat these words to yourself, **"Only small steps to cross the pond ..... (insert your name here)."**

Break down your long-term goal into five smaller chunks that will help you to achieve your journey, and see success gradually. These goals can be anything from clearing your wardrobe of all the old clothes that are too big for you, yet you save them in case you need them in the future, through to clearing your cupboards of all the sugary and fatty snacks you rely on when you get bored or fancy a small bite to nibble on.

Before you start, write down what will happen if you do not take action or commit today?

First Point of Action (including date to be completed)
Result:
Purpose:

Second Point of Action (including date to be completed)
Result:
Purpose:

Third Point of Action (including date to be completed)
Result:
Purpose:

Forth Point of Action (including date to be completed)

Result:
Purpose:

Fifth Point of Action (including date to be completed)
Result:
Purpose:

Q. How long will it take for you to achieve your goal?

The length it takes you to reach your goal is wholly dependent on how committed you are. The truth of it is that you are not just carrying out a programme but changing your life, and changing the way you think about how you look after your body, therefore the programme itself can take as long as it takes until you start seeing results – but this lifestyle change will last forever. Remember this change process will be hard, there is no doubt about it, however, the feelings of accomplishment and success far outweigh any pain encountered on your journey.

Achievers recognise why they want something and set out to achieve it, no matter what gets in their way. They understand the concept that "there is no failure only feedback" and this is a great belief to hold on to as it allows you to always grow and improve. You might not get the perfect result you want, but you will get a result. Based upon the result you achieve, you can then learn the appropriate lessons and go again.

Although seemingly tempting to considerably reduce your calorie intake in an effort to lose weight fast, you shouldn't aim to lose more than two pounds a week – although initially you may lose slightly more due to your body getting rid of water as well as fat. In the long term though, a weight loss of more than two pounds a week means you'll have to reduce calories excessively – and ultimately, this will make it even harder to shift those unwanted pounds as well as making failure more likely. Losing more than

Chapter One

two pounds a week can also play havoc with your digestion, and extreme weight loss may result in some people having saggy skin, something I presume you would want to avoid.

Therefore a delicate balance between reducing your calorie intake and cutting it drastically can be a fundamental segment to aid you in cutting those unwanted pounds and leaving you with the body you desire.

At two pounds a week, here is an idea of how long you can expect it to take you to lose weight...

1/2 Stone	5wks @ 1lb a Week	3 wks @ 2lb a Week
1 Stone	12 wks @ 1lb a Week	6 wks @ 2lb a Week
2 Stone	26 wks @ 1lb a Week	13 wks @ 2lb a Week
3 Stone	40 wks @ 1lb a Week	20 wks @ 2lb a Week
4 Stone	54 wks @ 1lb a Week	27 wks @ 2lb a Week
5 Stone	68 wks @ 1lb a Week	34 wks @ 2lb a Week
6 Stone	82 wks @ 1lb a Week	41 wks @ 2lb a Week
7 Stone	96 wks @ 1lb a Week	48 wks @ 2lb a Week
8 Stone	110 wks @ 1lb a Week	55 wks @ 2lb a Week
9 Stone	124 wks @ 1lb a Week	62 wks @ 2lb a Week

After seeing the rate at which you can potentially lose weight, whilst exercising and changing your nutritional balance, why not give yourself some markers to try to reach at different intervals throughout the year? Below you'll find a table to fill out, including dates, current weights and weights aimed for so that you can not only record where you are but also keep tabs on whether you are on track to reaching your goal.

Start by setting out a plan, dating when you will weigh yourself. Perhaps weekly, every two weeks or every month, whichever suits you. Remember this is your plan and it must fit in with your life if it is to work.

After that, simply refer to the chart above and set realistic goals for a weight that you would like to be on each of these dates. This will give you and your mind something to work towards. Remember to be realistic as the idea is to achieve your goals and feel great about it, definitely not the other way around.

On the required date, weigh yourself to see whether you have achieved your target. The final column is for you to note whether or not you have reached your goal.

Finally, and most importantly, when you have reached your goal, reward yourself.

Date
Goal Weight
Weigh in
+/-

Remember, when rewarding yourself, don't automatically think of something that you are not allowed, or that you are avoiding, such as sweet or fatty foods like pastries. Instead, how about treating yourself to something you do not often do such as a massage, or a manicure, or a new item of clothing that you have always wanted. There is more than one way of treating yourself. Remember to focus on the new you, the person you want to be. If you do so, you are already on the road to success.

What Can Trip You?

Now that you have set your goal, it is good to know what kind of things can get in your way, or trip you up, so that you can avoid them. If you're the kind of person who enjoys snacking on unhealthy treats, only stock your shelves with the healthy treats your body deserves when you do your food shopping. You can't eat what is not there! If there is a lot of junk food in the house that you are vulnerable to, ask the members of the house to put them somewhere you rarely go, or get rid of them altogether. Another idea is to put a lock on the cupboard, as every step you put between you and the foods you really don't want to eat, the easier it is to avoid eating them. Each physical barrier you put in place also creates a psychological barrier as to open a cupboard or reach up to a high shelf, you have to first think, "I want to open the cupboard," or, "I want to reach the shelf." Each such thought presents another opportunity for you to show your strength, and to just say "no."

There are going to be times within any programme when you may be tempted to slip back into your old bad habits, so you need to plan ahead. If you're the kind of person who is good at making excuses about why not to go to the gym, then make sure there is a good reason why you are going, perhaps a friend meeting you there or a reminder of the pain you were causing yourself before you took the first big step towards losing weight. Routine is important. Remember to stay positive and to focus on the benefits of losing weight — for your appearance, for your health — a good knowledge of your goals will help you here, but don't stress the negatives, as these will create a barrier between you and the weight loss you desire.

Write out three things that often got in your way in the past, or you can see preventing you doing what you intend to do. When you know what they are, you can avoid them.

1._____

2._____

3._____

"fat mind, fat body"

Chapter Two

Nutrition

Introduction

Congratulations on working your way through the first part of the book. You are now one step closer to massively changing your life forever.

Before moving on with this segment, a common misconception is that eating the correct food is more expensive than eating pre-packed fatty foods. I want to quash this from the start. It is not the case, so this is simply an excuse, and one often used by those who are experiencing weight issues. Sure, buying fresh vegetables from the most expensive supermarket is going to be more expensive than buying a family-sized lasagne from the frozen section, however, having eaten healthy food for most of my life, I know there is no real reason why it shouldn't cost the same as not-so-healthy food, if not less. Look for local vegetable markets where produce is bought wholesale and sold on at a much lower mark up than in the major supermarkets. Many of these markets also have bulk buy offers on bags of fruit and vegetables.

Another common misconception is that cooking fresh food takes a lot of time, with many people saying they don't have time to prepare anything other than a ready-meal. But, there are many meal options, such as stir-fries and wholesome soups, which require only a low level of cooking skill and can be ready in less than 20 minutes.

So, by now you will have a clear view of how you intend to lose the weight and the steps you are going to take to achieve your desired outcome. This chapter will educate you to be aware of what you are really eating, instead of what you think you are eating, along with giving tips and advice on ways you can adapt your current eating patterns into your new nutritional life. By the end of this chapter, you will not only understand the quality and quantity of different foods, but the reasons behind why you should avoid or approach certain foods. Remember that all of the advice given is just one set of ideas, and some of the concepts may work for you and not for others, and vice versa. Your weight loss is deeply personal to you, and no two people will have the same experience.

But before we move on to the nutritional aspect, it's important to revisit the importance of choice. Choice is the power to say either "yes" or "no" and your choice is going to be the deciding factor when it comes to adapting your lifestyle to one that positively supports your body, or one that negatively withdraws your ability to function effectively, to lose the weight, and to reach your goals. How you lose weight is personal to you, so the following is meant as a guide, offering varying levels of advice to cater for those who just want a few simple, general instructions and ideas, all the way through to those who want a more detailed and hands-on approach. This is not to suggest that you should not be dedicated or committed, but to recognise the fact that different people require different types of advice in order to succeed.

How Many Calories Am I Meant to Eat?

Essentially, the average intake of calories per day or the EAR (Estimated Average Requirements) stated by the UK Department of Health, show that women should consume around 1940 calories and men around 2550 calories per day. However, these figures are not going to be sufficient for everyone as there are a great many variations depending on lifestyle and other factors. But, there is another quick method that can help to establish the daily calorie intake needed for any individual based on body weight. The method uses your current body weight and a multiplier to determine your calorie needs.

Fat loss = 10 calories per lb of bodyweight

"fat mind, fat body" ───────────────────────────

> Maintenance = 13 calories per lb of bodyweight
> Weight gain: = 15 calories per lb of bodyweight

This calculation is a fast and easy way to establish your individual calorific intake, but the drawback is that it does not take into account your body composition or your daily level of activity. For example, if you are a highly active person, you may require far more calories than this formula indicates. A useful rule of thumb is that for every day you exercise for one hour at a moderate intensity (the level at which you can just about still talk), add 400 calories, or for one hour at a high intensity (the level at which talking becomes impossible), add 600 calories. If you don't exercise for a complete hour, divide 60 by the number of minutes you do exercise for, and then divide the calorie additions by this amount. Alternatively, search the internet for a list of popular exercises and the number of calories each one burns per hour depending on your body weight.

As the composition of the body is not taken into account in the above formulae, they may overestimate the requirement for anyone with a higher percentage of body fat. It is down to the individual's perception of the results given in comparison to the recommended daily amount to establish a suitable answer to the question of overall intake. The formulae are tools rather than rules. A more accurate but rather fiddlier way to work out your calorie needs is given below.

First you need to calculate your Basal Metabolic Rate (BMR) – the calories your body needs for energy balance at rest and then times it by a multiplier.

If you don't know your lean body weight:

Women: BMR = 655 + (9.6 times weight in kg) + (1.8 times height in cm) - (4.7 times age in years)

Men: BMR = 66 + (13.7 times weight in kg) + (5 times height in cm) - (6.8 times age in years)

Remember, there are 14lbs to a stone, 2.2lbs to a kg, and 1 inch to 2.54cm.

To work out your lean body weight from your body fat percentage, find out your total weight and times this by your body fat percentage divided by 100.

If you know your lean body weight:

BMR = 370 + (21.6 times lean body weight in kg)

Next you need to multiply your BMR by your level of physical activity from the following chart:

Little to no exercise	BMR x 1.2
Light exercise (1–3 days per week)	BMR x 1.375
Moderate exercise (3–5 days per week)	BMR x 1.55
Heavy exercise (6–7 days per week)	BMR x 1.725
Very heavy exercise (twice per day)	BMR x 1.9

To lose weight effectively in a way that can be easily maintained, you should aim for around 500-1000 calories less than this amount through a combination of both diet and exercise.

Q. How does your intake compare to these recommendations?

Tip. Search online for a food and calorie guide to compare your amounts.

Take a moment now to work out how many calories you will need to consume in a day to help towards succeeding in your goal of weight loss, bearing in mind that it takes around 3500 calories to burn one pound of fat.

Be realistic; remember it takes small steps to cross the pond.

Meal Size and Hunger Signals

For most of us, it's common to eat three meals a day, normally breakfast, lunch and dinner, as a matter of habit. Consuming three meals a day is sufficient and this number should not be exceeded unless you choose to have smaller meals more regularly. When eating three meals each day, it's important that two of them should be light as this allows your body to function at its optimum throughout the day. Large meals make big demands on the digestive organs, using much of your blood supply to break down the food in your stomach, which limit's the amount available to nurture the brain, preventing it from working efficiently. This will in turn lead to you having a lack of energy and feeling disinclined to work at your best. For this reason, if you're dealing with some work or an activity that requires a lot of concentration, it's better to conduct it after a light meal rather than a larger one. Larger meals also cause fluctuations in your hormone levels, again leading to a feeling of tiredness and a lack of concentration. This will also make it more difficult to exercise and more likely that you'll make poor food choices, so large meals can be counterproductive to your weight loss goals.

"Never eat more than you can lift."
- Miss Piggy

If the job you do requires a high level of physical effort then restricting the size of your meals is still important, but for different reasons. A key point to keep in mind is that physical work, like exercise, actually prevents digestion. If you eat large meals because of the type of work you do, then it is possible that you will wear yourself out due to hard work retarding digestion, and with the weakened digestion, fewer nutrients are digested from the food. With this in mind, people who have to work hard either physically or mentally throughout the day, or exercise a lot, are advised to eat a hearty meal after the day's work rather than before or during to ensure optimum efficiency, both in terms of fuelling their brain and in gaining maximum nutrition from the food that they eat.

The body's metabolism and internal activities also slow down during the hours of rest, and even more so during sleep. If you consume a heavy meal immediately before you retire for the evening, it will inevitably leave you feeling uncomfortable in the morning, as the food will not have digested well during your hours of sleep. Eating large meals before bed will also affect your sleep patterns, leading to you waking up tired and grumpy, and therefore making you less likely to follow a healthy eating and exercise plan. To avoid this uncomfortable feeling and to get a good night's rest, it is advised to eat at least two hours prior to going to sleep to allow your body time to efficiently digest the food you consume.

The human body is built on a process of natural pulses and hormone fluctuations called your circadian rhythm. It's a rhythm that adapts to regular practices; therefore setting your meal times at regular intervals is recommended as this facilitates your body's natural rhythms. A regular interval between meals is also conducive to health in general as the body works best when in sync with the natural circadian rhythm. To help you plan the timing of your meals, there should be a period of between four and a half to five hours between each meal, as it takes this long to fully digest the food you eat. Stomach digestion is only the beginning of the digestion process and this alone takes between two to five hours depending on what has been eaten, as well as the activity you do.

Q. At what times can you have meals to ensure you gain the most out of your digestive system?

Breakfast

"Breakfast like a king, lunch like a queen, dinner like a pauper."

The above saying makes good nutritional sense but clearly, and after reading this chapter, this is something that is highly dependent on each and everybody's individual lifestyles. A heavy breakfast is very common in England and America but on the European continent, a very light breakfast is much more the norm with a cup of coffee and a single bread roll being a favourite morning meal for the average Parisian. To eat enough to steal your brain away is a poor way to begin the day for anyone, and skipping breakfast is an equally poor idea as breakfast kick-starts your metabolism for the day ahead, increasing the number of calories you will burn off throughout your day.

It may not suit you to breakfast like a king but in terms of determining how much to eat in the morning it's worth noting that your body and brain will function much more efficiently on a breakfast of either fruit, cereal, toast, or a glass of milk than on eggs, fried potatoes or bread, or just coffee, which is not an uncommon breakfast. But, as stated earlier, it all depends on your lifestyle, time commitments and your personal daily routine. Take into consideration the concept of increasing your metabolism by eating smaller meals throughout the day, if possible, so that your body is always slowly working towards breaking down food, leading to you burning a few extra calories that can soon add up.

Slow digesting, low sugar foods also provide a steady stream of energy compared to high sugar foods that provide only short-term energy boosts. Many popular breakfast cereals are very high in sugar, so look out for those that are low in sugar (below 5g per 100g) and contain a significant amount of fibre (more than 3g per 100g). Good examples of slow digesting breakfast foods are porridge oats, high fibre bran, and various wheat biscuits. You can also add fibre to your morning meal by adding fresh fruit and nuts.

If you are going to have a cooked breakfast, consider poaching your eggs rather than frying them to reduce the fat content, using leaner cuts of bacon with the fat trimmed off rather than sausages – or use low fat sausages which are available in many supermarkets – and mushrooms which can be stir-fried with just a light touch of olive oil. Remember, the key to sticking to a healthy eating plan is variety so mix your meals up from one day to the next and keep things interesting.

Portion size...

What size of plate do you serve your meal on? As humans, we do not like to see an empty space on a plate so we feel obliged to fill it. Think about this for a moment, and then consider whether you could eat from a smaller plate or bowl. Filling the space on a large plate often leads to eating more than you actually need but with a smaller plate, even if you fill it, you still reduce the amount you eat.

If a larger plate is your only option, consider using the inner rim of the plate as a guide to portion size rather than the whole plate itself. And before deciding whether or not to have seconds, you should wait for around 20 minutes, as this is the amount of time it takes for your brain to acknowledge hunger signals when your stomach releases the hormone leptin to signal that you are full. Eating more slowly allows more time for your brain to realise that you actually don't need anything else to eat, whereas eating quickly can lead to making the assumption that you're still hungry, which may not actually be true. Similarly, consuming a glass of water whilst you eat gives your body longer to respond to the signals your brain sends.

Another excellent tip when preparing your daily meal is to use one handful, piled no higher than an inch, as a portion measure for carbohydrate ingredients (rice, potatoes, grains), a palm-full for the meat portion, and two handfuls for the vegetable portion of the meal.

Consider thinking about your weight loss goals whilst you are eating and focus on all that you wish to achieve; concentrate on your breathing and finish what is in your mouth before consuming the next forkful. Concentrate on the texture of the food and its flavour, and enjoy what you eat by not rushing it down. Avoid watching TV whilst you eat, as this will distract your brain from registering the hunger signals your body is sending to tell you that you are full.

Daily Nutritional Balance

The amount of food you eat in a day will inevitably have an outcome on your individual weight gain or weight loss, but it's also important to consider the types of food you eat. Your diet must be balanced and varied to ensure your body receives all of the nutrients it needs to work at its optimum.

The list below gives the percentages of each food type in a daily diet that will provide the best balance.

- **Carbohydrate foods – 33 per cent**

This group includes bread, pasta, cereals, and potatoes. Aim to consume four to five portions each day.

- **Fruit and vegetables – 33 per cent**

Aim to consume at least five portions to achieve your "5-a-day"!

- **Dairy products – 15 per cent**

This group includes milk, cheese etc.. Aim to consume three portions daily.

- **Protein foods – 12 per cent**

This group includes meat, fish, tofu and all other vegetarian "meat-free" alternatives. Aim to consume two to three portions each day.

- **Fats and sugars – 7 per cent or <u>one</u> portion**

This group includes all fatty foods and high sugar treats such as cakes, pastries, potato crisps, sweets, and fizzy drinks.

Of course, it's all very well knowing how many portions of what type of food you need during a day but how do you measure how much is in a portion?

Meat: When deciding on different portion sizes for meats, if you consider the piece of meat to be around the size of a pack of cards, you would be about right.

Fruit and vegetables: Many different food types measure their food portions in the form of cups, where one cup equals one portion. This is also the case when it comes to fruit and vegetables, although they can't just be poured into a measuring cup like pasta or rice. For example, a fist is around the same size as a cup, therefore a fist-sized apple would equal one portion.

"fat mind, fat body"

To help stick to the correct portion sizes, visualise your goals as you are eating and associate each plate of food with something positive like a favourite song or place. This way, you very soon won't even notice the reduced portion sizes, but you will notice the weight dropping from your waist and hips, and you will see how much closer you are to the you that you want to be.

Once you have established the portions you need to eat throughout the day to achieve a balanced diet, the task is now understanding how to split the portions up accordingly on your plate. There are two ways of looking at this, either via **food groups** or via **types of food**.

Food groups should be separated as follows:

    1/3 Carbohydrate
    1/3 Protein
    1/3 Fat

This may sound like a large amount of fat, but when broken down to the fat found in certain meats, and the fats your food may be cooked in, it balances out very quickly. It's important not to automatically associate fat with being "bad" as not all fats are equal – more on this later.

Food types provide a more intuitive method of breaking down your requirements. For example, fruit and vegetables, meat, and grains. Food types should be broken down as follows:

    1/2 plate filled with fresh vegetables and/or fruit
    1/4 plate with whole grains
    1/4 plate with lean meat

This distribution will contribute to achieving the essential balance of nutrients; including the various vitamins and minerals you need for a healthy diet.

Carbohydrates

Carbohydrates are one source of energy that the body gains from food. They can be readily converted into glucose, a simple type of sugar, transported and used around the body. Glucose is transported via your blood and taken into cells to be converted into energy. The pancreas gland in your abdomen secretes the hormone insulin that controls the uptake of glucose by your cells, and any excess is converted into glycogen, which is stored in the liver or as fat, triglycerides, around the body.

Consuming an insufficient amount or over indulging in carbohydrates can cause fluctuations in the body's sugar and energy levels, leaving you feeling either energetic for a short period of time followed by a sudden feeling of tiredness, or moody and frustrated. When your body needs more energy, the pancreas secretes a second hormone called glucagon. This hormone converts the glycogen back into glucose, which is then released into your bloodstream for your cells to use. Carbohydrates come in two basic forms, **complex carbohydrates** and **simple carbohydrates.**

Complex carbohydrates...

Complex carbohydrates, otherwise known as starchy carbohydrates, can be found in both natural and refined foods but are generally found in higher quantities in whole grains. They are broken down into glucose more slowly than simple carbohydrates, and therefore supply a gradual stream of energy throughout the day, creating a lower peak in insulin levels. This should prevent the sudden feeling of tiredness and subsequent desire for sugary foods commonly experienced with simple carbohydrates and foods high in sugar.

Natural sources of complex carbohydrates, including foods such as barley and oats, are less likely to rot your teeth than simple carbohydrates and refined sugars, also providing greater satiety, keeping you feeling fuller for longer and in turn, less likely to make poor food choices.

Listed below are some common sources of complex carbohydrates:

- Barley

- Bran

- Whole grains

- Beans

- Brown rice

- Chickpeas

- Lentils

- Nuts and seeds

- Oats

Refined foods can also give the body a good supply of carbohydrate. Sources can be found in many foods that have been processed, but they are generally less beneficial to your health than unprocessed foods. For example, white pasta contains refined starches, as the machinery processing removes the husk, or brown segment, of the grain that is left intact in whole grain pasta. This provides a finer texture and prolongs the shelf life of the product but it also removes important nutrients, such as B vitamins, fibre, iron, and other vitamins and minerals.

The more refined the carbohydrate, the faster the glucose is released into your bloodstream. This can cause peaks and drops in your blood sugar level, and less stable energy levels in the body which in turn can lead to an enhanced risk of poor food choices and exercise habits.

Listed below are some common sources of refined starches:

• Mashed potatoes

• Many popular cereals

• Wholemeal (notice the difference between wholemeal and whole grain)

• White bread

• White pasta

• White rice

Simple carbohydrates...

Simple carbohydrates are often seen as the "bad carbs" and are also known as sugars, having been broken down and then reformed to produce sweet products. However, they can exist in both a natural and reformed form with the natural kind found mostly in fruit and vegetables such as apples, melons and bananas. Simple carbohydrates are often added to food products to increase their sweetness, but foods containing lots of added sugar are also high in calories so when trying to lose weight, these foods should be avoided. Although both simple and complex carbohydrates in their natural form can contribute towards long-term good health, complex carbohydrates provide better appetite control and sustained energy levels than simple carbohydrates.

Listed below are some examples of foods containing simple sugars:

- Biscuits, cakes and pastries

- Chocolate

- Honey and jams

- Jellies

How much do I need?

The total amount of carbohydrate you consume in a day can affect the way in which your body behaves and is a key factor in a healthy diet as too much sugar or total carbohydrate can lead to the onset of Type II diabetes. In theory, we should get around half of our energy through eating carbohydrates, with a large percentage in the form of complex carbohydrates which are unrefined and low in calories, such as grains, whole cereals, and vegetables. Your aim should be to consume around five or six servings of grain and cereal each day, three or four servings of vegetables, and two servings of fruit, although not all carbohydrates are equal in their servings. Refined sugars should take up no more than 11 per cent of your daily diet and are best avoided when trying to lose weight.

Tip: Read the labels on packets and products containing more than 15g of sugar per 100g should be avoided and replaced with those containing less than 5g per 100g.

People worry about eating too many carbohydrates when on a diet as they are convinced that carbohydrates directly make them fat. Of course there is a balance between eating excess carbohydrates and eating enough to give you the energy you need to carry out the exercise you intend to do to lose weight. Although low-carb diets have had a lot of publicity, gram for gram carbohydrates contain less calories than fat, protein, and alcohol. And remember, low-carb diets are notoriously difficult to follow for any but the briefest period of time. In the appropriate amount, starchy carbohydrates can be a vital instrument within your toolkit for success.

1g of carbohydrate contain 3.75 calories.

1g of protein contain 4 calories.

1g of fat contain 9 calories.

1g of alcohol contain 7 calories.

Very often, it is the way a carbohydrate foodstuff is prepared for eating that makes the difference between it being considered a "good" or "bad" element in a healthy diet. Many high sugar (simple carbohydrate) foods are also prepared by cooking in fat, such as chips and roast vegetables, which changes the overall nutritional value of the food, leading us to believe that the food is "bad" when it is in fact the cooking method that causes the change in the nutrient profile.

"An apple a day keeps the doctor away."

Different types of carbohydrate can aid your diet as well as your health. By consuming starchy foods such as whole grain bread, whole grain pasta and other complex carbohydrates that are rich in fibre, you also benefit your digestive health, help to control your appetite by keeping hunger at bay, and prevent some food from being reabsorbed in your bowel, thus reducing your calorie intake.

As sugar and starch are found in both healthy and "unhealthy" foods, it is both the type and the amount of carbohydrate you eat that is very important for your wellbeing and achieving your weight loss goals. Now, you are probably wondering how much carbohydrate you eat in your daily diet? In order to know this, you must first know how much carbohydrate is in the food you eat.

How much carbohydrate is contained in different foods?

One slice of bread (1oz): 15g carbohydrate

One small apple (4oz): 15g carbohydrate

One medium apple (6oz): 25g carbohydrate

One spoon of sugar (1 tbsp): 15g carbohydrate

One small baked potato (3oz): 15g carbohydrate

One large baked potato (12oz): 60-70g carbohydrate

Cooked spaghetti pasta (1 Cup): 40g carbohydrate

Glycemic Index

Another useful concept to bear in mind – and empower you on your mission to lose weight and achieve the body of your dreams – is the Glycemic Index, or GI for short. This is a measure of how many certain foods containing carbohydrates raise your blood sugar levels. Foods that break down quickly and release glucose rapidly have a high GI, and foods that break down and release glucose slowly have a low GI. The GI level is calculated by comparing the amount of glucose released in the two hours after consuming a food with a standard, usually table sugar or sometimes white bread. A low GI is any food with a GI score below 55 and a high GI is any food with a score above 70. Higher blood sugar means more insulin is released, making it more likely that you will store fat, rather than burn it off. As your metabolism of fat slows down, the number of calories you need to consume to achieve an energy balance is reduced.

A recent concept called Glycemic Load (GL) has updated GI to account for the differing levels of carbohydrates found in different foods. High dietary glycemic loads have been associated with an increased risk of developing Type II diabetes in several large studies. In the Nurses' Health Study, women with the highest dietary glycemic loads were 37 per cent more likely to develop the condition over a six year period than women with the lowest dietary glycemic loads. The results of the Health Professionals Follow-up Study, which monitored male health professionals over six years, were similar.

Calculating Glycemic Load...

$$\frac{GI \times \underline{available\ carbohydrates}}{100} \text{ (total carbohydrate minus fibre)}$$

In order to make it easier for you to use this information, I have included a list of common substitutions you can make using a food's GL below:

• Chips / root vegetable alternatives: Carrots, yams, cassava, parsnips are all better than sweet potatoes, in turn sweet potatoes are better than white potatoes.

"fat mind, fat body"

- Cereals: Bran, fruit and fibre, shredded wheat, and porridge, have a lower GL than most alternatives. Adding fruit with skin improves the food's GL.

- Fruits: Lychees, raisins, and sultanas are not as good as other fruits.

- Grains: Whole grains, basmati rice, and black rice are better than other varieties.

- Bread: Rye bread and gluten free are better than whole grain, and whole grain is better than white, brown and wholemeal.

- Takeaways: Chicken chow mein, balti dishes (without too much added oil), and chicken breast kebab with salad, are better than most other alternatives.

- Desert: Carrot cake and banana cake (with coconut flour), plain muffins, and nut bars, are better than most alternatives.

An important factor to bear in mind when choosing foods by GL is that this method doesn't take into account the fat content of the food, so be careful to avoid foods high in fat (greater than 20g per 100g), and saturated fat (greater than 5g per 100g).

Tip: Search online for a list of common foods and their GI/GL values.

Remember when substituting foods to tell yourself about the benefits the foods you are choosing will bring and how much closer to achieving your goals it will take you. Use positive words and imagery to reinforce your positive food choices.

Q. Do you consume many sugary foods?

Chapter Two

Q. Do you mainly consume high GL or low GL carbohydrates?

Q. What could you substitute for your high GL choices?

Q. What foods do you enjoy the most from the low GL list?

Write an alternative-shopping list, substituting low GL foods for your normal higher GL choices. Do this for every item you consider worth changing. Imagine how much better you will feel and how much further towards your goal these choices will help you reach. Make sure that your options remain realistic.

Shopping List:

_____

_____

_____

_____

_____

_____

Fats

Although it is not completely understood, or accepted in most diets, fat is an essential part of our nutritional balance. Fats can provide a source of concentrated energy along with being used in the transportation of vital nutrients around the body. It also allows for the digestion and metabolism of the fat soluble vitamins A,

D, E and K, needed for hormone construction, growth, eyesight, appetite, taste, immunity, bone health, and clotting amongst other functions.

Misunderstandings concerning fat generally revolve around the type of fat that is consumed and the volume. Every part of a human's nutritional consumption must be balanced so as not to lead to overloading a certain area, be it fats, carbohydrates, or any other element of the diet. At the end of the day, we all need a certain level of fat to maintain healthy skin and hair at the very least, but also for tissue repair, and more importantly, for protecting the internal organs and preventing excessive loss of body heat.

Outlined below are the main types of fat along with an explanation of the differences between them. Remember that fat is important for your overall health, but the type of fat consumed can have a significant impact in terms of helping you to reach your goals.

Trans fat...

Trans fats are found in processed foods, most notably hydrogenated vegetable oils (most cooking oils except virgin olive oil). There has been a push towards trans fats in foods due to companies seeking to replace saturated fats, and the associated adverse health effects, but, unfortunately, recent research suggests trans fats are as bad for our health, if not worse, as they raise bad cholesterol levels (LDL cholesterol) in the same way as saturated fat. Trans fats can be found in hard margarines that are formed by the 'hydrogenation' of vegetable oils. This process increases the melting point of the fat, meaning that it not only has a longer shelf-life but it is also great for baking. Of course, the flip side of this benefit is that it is harmful to your health. Trans fats are used because they are cheap, add bulk to products, and have a neutral flavour. Avoid foods cooked in non virgin cooking oils and also margarines that are not "trans fat free" as trans fats are not essential in the human diet. However, it must be remembered that replacing trans fats with saturated fats can still lead to health problems.

"The trans fats found in food containing hydrogenated vegetable oil are harmful and have no known nutritional benefits. They raise the type of cholesterol in the blood that increases the risk of coronary heart disease. Some evidence suggests that the effects of these trans fats may be worse than saturated fats. It's important to try to eat less of both saturated fat and trans fats." - The Food Standards Agency.

Current recommendations are that we should consume less than two per cent of our daily calories in the form of trans fats, and health authorities worldwide recommend that consumption of trans fats be reduced to trace amounts.

Saturated Fat...

Unlike trans fats, saturated fat is essential, but only in small amounts. Saturated fats help us to make hormones that regulate the processes within our body and provide rigidity to cell membranes, preventing them from collapsing. However, saturated fat is commonly consumed in too large an amount, a fact raised by the National Nutrition and Dietary Survey in 2010. We need no more than 10 per cent of our daily calories from saturated fat. Too much saturated fat can be dangerous as it can raise LDL ("bad") cholesterol which can in turn can lead to the arteries carrying blood to your heart becoming clogged up, a process known by the medical term of atherosclerosis. The biggest UK killer is coronary heart disease; in 2006 there were around 126,000 deaths from coronary heart disease in the UK. The most common cause of coronary heart disease is too much harmful LDL cholesterol in the blood − without being overly technical, not all forms of LDL

"fat mind, fat body"

are equal, but both saturated and trans fats raise the worst types of LDL. Excessive amounts of saturated fat are often found in animal fats and also in many "ready meals" as like trans fats, they increase the shelf-life of the product as they are more stable in processing than mono and poly unsaturated fats. Too much saturated fat, like sugar, can also affect insulin levels.

Listed below are some common products that contain saturated fats:

- Meat

- Butter

- Cream

- Cheese

- Ready meals

- Egg yolks

As with trans fats, health authorities worldwide recommend that consumption of saturated fats be reduced due to its negative effect on health. A simple way to reduce your intake is to consume leaner meats and reduce the amount of processed meats in your diet, such as mince, burgers, and sausages. Other options are to try replacing mince with lean steak mince, eating low fat sausages, or try "Quorn" products instead of meat. It is also worth bearing in mind that non-processed white meats such as chicken, turkey and fish are generally lower in saturated fat than red meat, particularly if you remove the skin from the chicken first. A good alternative to full fat milk is skimmed milk (less than one per cent fat), and you could try having soya milk instead. Double cream can be replaced with single cream, or lower fat alternatives such as reduced fat crème fresh. Or, if making a sauce, choose vegetable based sauces instead of creamy ones, and use a blended mixture of low fat cheese and skimmed milk as a cream substitute in savoury recipes such as a carbonara. Eggs contain a lot of essential nutrients, vitamins, and minerals so they should not be completely eliminated from your diet, but ensure you eat fewer than seven a day to limit the effect on your cholesterol levels.

The way you cook your food can also affect the fat content. By grilling or steaming food instead of cooking it in oil, you can heavily reduce the fat content, and this applies to all foods, not just meats. For example, potatoes have little or no fat content until they are deep fried, adding lots of saturated fat to the food. If you do cook in fat, think about the type of fat you use. Avoid butter and lard, and use oils such as olive oil instead. Non-stick pans can also help to reduce the amount of oil you need to use in cooking, and you could also start using spices to add flavour to your food rather than adding fat. Remember, saturated fat is a barrier to your healthy weight loss goals.

Unsaturated Fat...

Unsaturated fats are generally liquid at room temperature. They are found predominantly in plant products and also in fish, particularly oily varieties like mackerel. There are two forms of unsaturated fat, polyunsaturated and monounsaturated, with examples of foods containing unsaturated fat including:

- Soybeans, sunflower, fish, and corn oils (polyunsaturated)

- Olive, peanut, and canola oils (monounsaturated)

The fatty acids found in unsaturated fat can't be manufactured by your body and therefore have to be consumed in the food you eat.

"fat mind, fat body"

Fatty acids are needed for energy production, helping to diffuse oxygen in the bloodstream, the production of haemoglobin, lowering high blood LDL cholesterol, raising levels of healthy cholesterol (HDL cholesterol), stabilising blood sugar levels, strengthening your immune system, and reducing water retention by assisting in sodium and water removal amongst many other functions. Substituting saturated fatty acids with unsaturated ones is a positive step towards achieving your weight loss goals.

Good sources of unsaturated fats include:

• Avocados (one quarter of an avocado contains 5g of unsaturated fat)

• Unsalted nuts (cashew, brazil, pecan, walnut)

• Seeds (pumpkin, sunflower, sesame)

• Virgin olive oil and other non-hydrogenated oils (three teaspoons provides your daily minimum requirements)

Omega-3 and omega-6 essential fatty acids are both types of unsaturated fat. They play an important role in the functions of the body that promote health and wellbeing. In particular, studies have shown that omega-3 fatty acids protect against heart disease and may also improve memory and concentration as high levels of DHA (docosahexaenoic acid, a type of omega-3) are found in the brain. Oily fish provides the best source of omega-3, and fresh fish are better than tinned.

Good sources of omega-3 fatty acids include:

• Salmon

• Tuna (avoid varieties stored in brine due to the salt content

- Trout

- Mackerel

- Sardines (avoid varieties stored in brine due to the salt content)

Current advice is to eat oily fish two to three times a week, and no more than once a week during pregnancy due to the level of heavy metals caused by sea pollution.

While oily fish is the best source of essential fatty acids, but other omega rich foods include:

- Corn oil

- Flaxseed oil

- Olive oil

- Nut oil

- Sunflower oil

As you now know, different fats provide different benefits for the human body, but all types of fat help to improve both the taste and odour of your food, along with helping to create a feeling of fullness after a meal. They are also essential in aiding the absorption of the fat-soluble vitamins (A, D, E and K) in the body. Many people consume too much total fat, as well as saturated fat, and as fat has a lot of calories this is one reason why many people are overweight.

Scientific studies have shown that rats given a choice of high fat food over a lower fat alternative will normally choose the high fat meal, this implies that fat may be addictive. So it is important

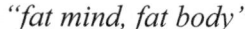

that you are aware of how much fat you actually need and that you reinforce your positive health choices with the techniques already discussed.

How much fat do I need?

Most people (in the UK) eat around 20 per cent too much saturated fat in relation to their Recommended Daily Allowance (RDA). Irrespective of the type of fat you are consuming, all fats contain nine calories per gram, so it is recommended that the average person should eat no more than 600 calories per day via their fat intake. This is based on 2000 calories per day diet whereby 30 per cent of the daily intake is made up of fat consumption. This works out to be around 65g per day of fat – an amount it's easy to go over in just one large meal, so you need to be careful.

Tell yourself that you don't desire those fatty foods you used to eat, but what you do desire is the new you, the you that you will achieve if you stick to your goals. Over time, you will find it easier and easier to make the right choices, the choices that will lead you to that new healthy body you desire and deserve.

As we have worked out, 65g of fat is around about sufficient for a day. This works out at around 22g per meal without trying to be too specific, remember that you may not always eat just one course per meal. Almost all labels on the food you eat can tell you the nutritional value of certain produce. Foods with more than 20g of total fat and 5g of saturated fat are considered high fat, and foods with 3g of total fat or 1.5g or less of saturated fat are considered low fat, so keep this in mind when considering your meal and snack options.

How much fat is contained in different foods?

A slice of French bread contains 1.4g of fat

A tablespoon of tartare sauce contains 8g of fat

1 oz of Brie contains 7.9g of fat

One whole large egg contains 5g of fat

A single chocolate chip cookie contains 2.2g of fat

1 teaspoon of regular butter has 3.8g of fat

3.5 oz of salami has 19.9g of fat

It can be helpful to keep a food diary of everything you eat for a week and to refer to the labels on the food you eat to calculate how much fat you are eating. You can then eliminate the foods highest in total fat and saturated fat or substitute them for healthier alternatives. Your weight loss is deeply personal to you and the act of keeping a diary in itself can help to make you more aware of how much food you are eating and may be another step forwards on the way to the new you. Remember, most people eat too much fat and therefore struggle to lose the weight.

Cut the bad fats and cut the waist size.

Q. How much total and saturated fat do you eat?

Q. Can you substitute lower fat alternatives?

Q. Can you use more unsaturated fats?

Write out a shopping list substituting lower fat and unsaturated fat alternatives in place of the unhealthier fats in your diet. Look at each replacement item and think of ways to describe it positively to yourself. For example, "I am going to use virgin olive oil rather than hydrogenated vegetable oil and it will help me lose weight, giving me the body I want."

Shopping List:

_____

_____

_____

_____

_____

Protein

Along with carbohydrates and fat, your body also needs protein. Protein is a nutrient that allows your body to function properly and maintain good health and all proteins are made up of different combinations of 20 compounds called amino acids, which come in two forms.

Essential amino acids: these cannot be made by the body and must be obtained from food.

Histine
Isoleucine
Leucine
Lysine
Methionine
Phenylalanine

Threonine
Tryptophan

Non-essential amino acids: these can be made by the body.

Alanine
Arginine
Asparagine
Aspartic acid
Cysteine
Glutamic acid
Glutamine
Glyceine
Proline
Serine
Tyrosine

Your body manufactures the 13 non-essential amino acids listed above but to function properly, the nine essential amino acids must also be made available to your body through dietary sources. Proteins are the building blocks of all life and are essential for the growth of cells and tissue repair, as well as enzyme and hormone formation. Protein malnutrition is very rare in the Western world as most people consume more protein than they require, but it is far more common in Africa and can lead to diseases such as kwashiorkor and in extreme cases eventually death.

The protein you eat helps to maintain and repair your body's tissue. It is found in almost every living cell and fluid. Depending on which amino acids link together, protein molecules form enzymes, hormones, muscles, organs and many other tissues in the body. Many of your hormones are made up of protein, and it is also used in the manufacturing of haemoglobin, found within the red blood cells that carry oxygen around your body. Protein is also used to manufacture antibodies that fight infection and disease and is integral to your body's blood clotting ability. Both children and adults need plenty of protein to grow and develop. Proteins are described as either complete or incomplete with complete proteins supplying adequate amounts of essential amino acids, and incomplete proteins supplying only a limited number of essential amino acids with others missing.

Both types can be found in different food groups with meat, eggs, and dairy products considered as complete proteins, supplying all of the essential amino acids needed, and vegetables, beans and other plant products considered as incomplete proteins. Common sources of protein are given below in two categories. The animal proteins contain all the essential amino acids and the plant proteins contain many, but not all, essential amino acids.

Animal Protein:

• Meat and poultry

• Fish

• Eggs

• Dairy products

Plant Protein:

• Legumes (peas, green beans)

• Cereals

• Beans

• Pulses

- Grains

- Nuts

- Seeds

- Soya products

- Vegetable protein foods (like Quorn or veggie mince)

If you do not eat meat, it is still possible to gain all of the essential amino acids your body needs through combining the different proteins available in plant based foods with non-meat animal proteins, such as milk and cheese, to make up the complete variety needed. Eating foods such as cereal with milk can help do this.

Vegans can also get their full protein requirement by mixing together the different vegetable sources consuming a mixture of beans, nuts, plants, soya, and seeds but this is more difficult and it may be useful to check the labels when planning such meals. Although meat has all of the essential amino acids you need, it is often high in saturated fat that you don't need, so it is recommended that you consume only two to three portions of red meat a weak (preferably lean) and use a mixture of non red meat and plant based protein sources to make up the rest of your diet.

How much do I need?

It is said that protein, unlike carbohydrate, should take up only around 10 to 15 per cent of your diet to meet the demands of your body, in relation to the recommended number of calories you need to consume in a day. With this in mind, a woman consuming 2000 calories per day and a man consuming 2500 calories per day would need at least 200 calories and 250 calories respectively from protein sources. In terms of weight, this works out at around 50g for women and 63g for men, but as a general guide, you should try to eat no more than around 1g of protein per kg of body weight. Eating excessive protein can cause a condition known as ketoacidosis, in which your blood's acidity is increased affecting the action of many enzymes and possibly in extreme cases leading to death, but this is not a common condition, as a diet of almost exclusively protein would need to be consumed.

However, it is evident that currently many people, if not most, eat more than the recommended 10 to 15 per cent, with the British Nutrition Foundation calculating the average adult intake to be 88g for men and 64g for women. But, the figures are overly generalised as the amount of protein required for normal health is variable depending on many factors, including body weight, age, physical activity, health condition, and environment amongst others. Generally, protein intake should be in equilibrium with protein loss. Protein is lost in urine, faeces, blood, sweat, skin, nails, and hair. When protein intake is less than protein loss, it is called negative protein balance, so in the reverse situation when protein intake is greater than protein loss, it is called positive protein balance. Ideally, a neutral protein balance should be attained in healthy adults.

For adults taking part in extreme exercise programmes such as elite athletes and bodybuilders, working out at least five days a week at a high intensity, the body's protein requirements may increase to around 0.7-1g per lb or 1.75g-2.2g per kg of lean body weight.

How much protein is contained in different foods?

Different types of food contain varying amounts of protein. Listed below are a variety of different sources and the amounts of protein they provide.

>One skinless chicken breast (130g): 41g protein.
>
>One small fillet steak (200g): 52g protein.
>
>One beef burger or pork sausage: 8g protein.
>
>One portion of poached skinless cod fillet (150g): 32g protein.
>
>Half a can of tuna: 19g protein.
>
>One portion of cheese (50g): 12g of protein.
>
>One medium egg: 6g of protein.
>
>150ml glass of milk: 5g of protein.
>
>One tablespoon of boiled red lentils (40g): 3g of protein.
>
>One portion of tofu (125g): 15g of protein.
>
>One slice medium wholemeal bread: 4g of protein.
>
>One slice medium white bread: 3g of protein.

Protein has one benefit in the diet that is much hyped by proponents of low-carb diets and this is that it can fill you up for longer than most other foods. Protein takes longer to digest, so this can lead to you eating fewer calories than with other food types, but, remember, many high protein foods are also high in fat, so choose healthier options as snacks to fill you up in-between meals; nuts, seeds, or low sugar grain based bars for example.

Q. Are you eating too much protein?

"fat mind, fat body"

Q. Can you think of healthier, leaner, alternatives to the protein you are eating?

Q. Are you eating two to three portions of oily fish a week?

Q. Are you consuming no more than two to three portions of lean red meat a week?

Q. Can you reduce the amount of processed, fatty, meat you eat?

Write out your shopping list, again substituting the healthier protein alternatives wherever possible. Reinforce the positive change you are making, ensuring that this is a viable option and it is sustainable.

Shopping List:

_____

_____

_____

_____

_____

Fibre

Fibre, also known as "roughage", is a part of your diet that is sourced solely from plants and cannot be digested by the human body. It is essentially a carbohydrate and found within the cell walls of many of the plants we eat. Although it can't be absorbed, and therefore provides no calories, fibre holds a very important role in the human diet as it helps to lower your blood cholesterol and control blood sugar levels, in turn helping to control your appetite. Fibre comes in many different forms, present in everything from rice and oats through to different types of fruit, with the only differences in types being their solubility.

Fibre passes through the body virtually unchanged, along with other digested food, until it arrives at the large intestine. The type of fibre consumed dictates the way in which it will aid the digestion process, with insoluble fibre helping food to pass through your bowel, preventing constipation and aiding the consistency of your stools. Fibre passes through the body quickly, taking with it the waste material unused by your body. This is important as it prevents toxins accumulating in the intestines which in turn helps to prevent diseases such as bowel cancer and irritable bowel syndrome.

Insoluble fibre...

The following foods are the main contributors to your insoluble fibre intake:

• Beans

• Brown rice

• Fruits with edible seeds

• Lentils

• Maize

- Most wholemeal products

Soluble fibre...

Soluble fibre contains gums and pectin. This type of fibre lowers cholesterol levels as the soluble fibre binds the cholesterol from food or from bile acids (made up of cholesterol), preventing it from being reabsorbed into the bloodstream. As the fibre cannot be digested, it is then eliminated as waste. Soluble fibre also controls and stabilises blood sugar levels by slowing down digestion and the sudden release of energy, especially from carbohydrates, into the bloodstream.

It can be found in all fruit and vegetables, but the following are rich sources:

- Apples

- Barley

- Citrus

- Guar gum

- Oats

- Pulses

- Strawberries.

How much do I need?

It is advised that an average adult should eat around 18g of fibre per day, but the current average is slightly below this at around 12g, meaning that the majority of us are not eating enough fibre. The biggest health effect comes from consuming mainly soluble fibre sources, but a diet that does not contain enough fibre of any type can lead to bowel irregularities and stomach discomforts. A food containing 6g of fibre per 100g or ml is considered to be a "high fibre" food but all sources of fibre should contain at least 3g fibre per 100g or ml to be of benefit to the body.

Q. Do you get enough fibre?

How much fibre is contained in different foods?

One bowl bran flakes (30g): 4.5g fibre.

One bowl fruit and fibre cereal (30g): 2.7g fibre.

One slice (28g) white bread: 0.8g fibre.

One slice (28g) wholemeal bread: 1.9g fibre.

One portion (80g) lentils: 1.5g fibre.

One orange (160g): 2.7g fibre.

One portion (80g) boiled cabbage: 1.7g fibre.

One portion penne pasta (90g dry weight): 2.3g fibre.

One portion whole-wheat pasta (90g dry weight): 9g fibre.

5-a-day

"fat mind, fat body"

One of the most essential elements of maintaining a healthy nutritional balance is ensuring that a high level of fruit and vegetables form part of the daily diet. For weight loss, fruit and vegetables are generally low in both fat and calories whilst being high in essential vitamins and minerals as well as fibre. Simply adding vegetables to your meal will leave you feeling fuller and lead to you consuming fewer calories at the same time. Fruit and vegetables can also be used as a great tool when used as substitutes in times of craving fatty/sugary foods.

Q. Do you currently eat you 5-a-day?

Since the turn of the millennium, government bodies have been trying to push the knowledge of getting your "5-a-day" and it has been scientifically proven that by carrying out this recommendation there are indeed fantastic health benefits to be had. These include reducing the risk of heart disease, Type II diabetes, and some cancers. Remember, fruits and vegetables are packed with vitamins and minerals such as vitamin C, folic acid, and potassium, in addition to being a fantastic source of fibre and antioxidants.

Even though people are aware of the benefits of adapting their diet, only one out of seven people actually make a change...are you one of them?

People looking for excuses as to why they fail to look after their body as efficiently as possible might say that they just do not have the time to stock their shelves on a day-to-day basis with fresh produce. This means we need to look for practical ways to make our shopping time as effective as possible, and to make sure the produce purchased lasts. To this end, why not buy canned, frozen, and juiced fruit and vegetables? These are items that will store for longer, allowing you to spend time on other things. Or, why not set aside one day of the week for fresh produce shopping, perhaps during the weekend. At the end of the day, one of the few things we all have in common is a 24 hour day, so if someone else can find the time, so can you!

Q. How can you introduce eating an extra piece of fruit into your daily routine?

Another concern many people have is the cost. People seem to be prepared to spend surprisingly little on something that is going to benefit them, yet if you compare the cost of an apple or banana to the cost of a chocolate bar or bag of crisps, it's actually the latter that represents an extortionate cost! The truth is that the piece of fruit is the more financially beneficial option, providing more nourishment for fewer calories. If the cost is still a genuine concern, purchase your fruit and vegetables at markets where they are often cheaper, and buy the options that are in season as the price is always going to be lower on items that are readily available. An added benefit of buying in season produce is that it will taste much nicer too.

Of course, a genuine excuse for avoiding fruit and vegetables is a genuine dislike of the taste. However, with the vast array of fruits and vegetables on the market today, it's difficult to believe that a dislike of everything that's on offer is a genuine excuse. There are so many textures and flavours available that it's just a matter of finding the ones you like and adapting them to your personal meal plan.

Tip: recipe books aimed at creating healthy family meals contain many ingenious ways of disguising vegetables for "fussy" eaters.

Q. Name three different fruits that you can include in your nutrition plan?

Q. Name three different vegetables that you can include in your nutrition plan?

"fat mind, fat body"

What can be considered as one portion of your 5-a-day?

1 apple, banana, pear, orange, or other similar sized fruit

2 plums, Satsuma oranges, kiwi fruit, or other similar sized fruit

1/2 a grapefruit or avocado

1 large slice of melon or fresh pineapple

3 heaped tablespoons of vegetables, beans or pulses

3 heaped tablespoons of fruit salad or stewed fruit

1 heaped tablespoon of raisins or sultanas

3 dried apricots

1 cup full of grapes, cherries or berries

1 dessert bowl of salad

1 150ml (small) glass of pure fruit juice

Remember, by simply increasing your fruit and vegetable intake, you are one step closer to achieving your goals.

The human body as a whole is composed of 30 per cent solids and 70 per cent water, with our blood consisting of 83 per cent water, bones 22 per cent water, and muscle 75 per cent water. Water, therefore, is the most important component of all complex living organisms. If we do not drink enough water throughout the day, the end result might be excess body fat, poor muscle tone, digestive complications, muscle soreness, and even water retention. Your body needs water to regulate body temperature and to provide the means for nutrients to travel to all of your organs. It's also water that transports oxygen to your cells, removes waste, makes you feel fuller, and protects your joints and organs.

As humans, we can go without food for almost a couple of months, but without water we may only last a couple of days, yet people still don't seem to drink enough, to the extent that many live in a dehydrated state. Even the smallest degree of water loss can impair physical and mental function and nutritionists have concluded that an overwhelming 80 per cent of us walk around most of the day in a state of dehydration.

Q. How much water do you drink each day?

Very often when we are feeling "thirsty", our first point of call may be a drink that actually causes more harm than good. Caffeinated drinks or alcohol can actually cause dehydration rather than counteract it, and in fact, your body is often dehydrated long before you actually experience a feeling of thirst. So with this mind, it is a good idea to drink water regularly throughout the day, even if your body is not telling you that you need it. Of course, even though it is the most efficient form of hydration, water isn't everybody's first tipple; therefore fruit juices, herbal/fruit teas and decaffeinated hot drinks can be an efficient alternative. If you feel unwilling or unable to switch from caffeinated drinks then don't worry, provided you have no more than one cup of standard strength tea within an hour or one cup of coffee within two hours, then the dehydration effect of the caffeine will be less than the hydration effect of the water in the cup.

The average amount of water needed by the human body is around two litres per day, comparable to around six to eight glasses, but this does not include during exercise or in hot weather, when needs will increase. A key indicator to a dehydrated body is the colour of your urine, the clearer the better. If your urine is a deep, dark colour, then you need to top up your water levels. Everyone is unique in terms of the amount of water their body requires but ensuring you manage at least two litres each day is a good start.

Q. What can you change to ensure that you drink more water during the day?

Water and weight loss...

There are many different forms of metabolism occurring in the body all of the time, but the one most people are interested in is the metabolism of fat. One of your liver's main concerns is converting fat into energy, along with helping the kidneys when they have too much to do. In order to work at their optimum, the kidneys need water. If the kidneys are deprived of water, the liver has to do their work in addition to its own, thereby reducing the efficiency of your body's fat metabolism. To aid your weight loss goals, it's essential that you are properly hydrated at all times.

As we have already discussed, water also naturally reduces your appetite. Making sure your water levels are topped up will reduce the chances of you snacking on those easy to prepare and quick to eat snacks as a lot of people confuse feeling thirsty with feeling hungry, leading to eating when really their body is telling them they should be drinking. When your body is dehydrated, your fat cells become harder to break down, so as a consequence, losing weight becomes harder when you're not drinking enough water.

Q. When was the last time you fancied something small to snack on and chose instead to have a glass of water?

Why not start today by replacing your snacks with water?

Cold water is better. It has been shown that colder water can be absorbed more quickly into the digestive system, but more importantly, it can increase the burning of calories. More calories are used in the process of heating the water in your stomach to get it to a sufficient temperature, thereby boosting your metabolism. Many of the above concepts, such as how much of what to eat or drink, all depend on your lifestyle, but following some of the basic principles mentioned will provide a good start. For a more personal structure, you may still need to consult a nutritionist.

Alcohol

We all enjoy a good drink, but most of us drink more than is good for our health and many of us drink in binges. "Binge drinking" used to mean drinking heavily over several days, but now the term refers to the heavy consumption of alcohol over a short period of time (just as binge eating means a specific period of uncontrolled eating). Today, the generally accepted definition of binge drinking is the consumption of five or more alcoholic drinks in a row by men and four or more alcoholic drinks by women, at least once in the past two weeks. Heavy binge drinking includes three or more binges over the two-week period. Research from the Department of Health shows that a man drinking five pints of alcohol a week consumes the same number of calories a year as someone who gets through 221 doughnuts.

Many people mistakenly think that alcohol is converted into fat, but in reality, the picture is much more complicated. Alcohol is used directly by the body as energy, providing seven calories per gram. This is used in preference to other fuel sources, so when your body is burning off alcohol it is not burning off fat. Most alcoholic drinks also contain excess amounts of sugar increasing the risk of developing Type II diabetes, and this sugar can also be stored as fat as the body is using the alcohol in the drink as its primary source of fuel. The sugar in the drink can also affect the body's insulin levels, causing a sudden peak followed by a drop, during which you are more likely to feel hungry and desire the type of foods that could derail your healthy eating plan. Excessive alcohol can also lead to psychological problems, problems with the skin, an increased risk of contracting certain cancers, as well as potentially leading to liver damage. Remember, your liver is the primary organ involved in the digestion of fat as well as the fat-soluble vitamins A, D, E, and K.

Whilst there are some things we can do to avoid a morning hangover, like drinking water before bed or taking milk thistle and silymarin supplements, there is nothing we can to do to avoid the negative effects of excess alcohol consumption on our appearance and waistline. It is therefore very important that you know how much alcohol you can have and stay healthy.

How much alcohol can I have?

The advice from the Department of Health is rather straightforward, but varies for men and women. Men can have a total of 21 units of alcohol a week or three to four units a day, whereas women can have 14 units of alcohol a week or two to three units a day. This is all well and good but many of you will now be asking; what is a unit of alcohol?

A unit of alcohol can be related to standard measures using the following chart:

Type of drink	**1 Alcoholic unit**
Beers (3.5 per cent proof)	Half a pint
Canned beer (5 per cent proof)	Half a can

Chapter Two

Wines (175ml glass, 12 per cent proof)   Half a glass
Wines (250ml glass, 12 per cent proof)   Third of a glass
Fortified wines (50ml glass)   One glass
Spirits (25ml glass)   One glass

The problem with this table, as with all tables, is that it can't cover every option available, so there is a formula you can use to work out how many units a drink contains given the volume in ml and the alcohol percentage.

$$\text{Alcohol units} = \frac{\text{volume in ml} \times \text{alcohol percentage}}{1000}$$

Q. Are you consuming too much alcohol?

A simple tip to reduce your alcohol intake is to have a soft drink in-between each alcoholic one. Another idea is to volunteer as the designated driver. Alternatively, low or non-alcohol drinks, such as the low alcohol beers and wines now stocked in many bars, provide healthier options, and you might be surprised by their taste.

Think of three ways you could reduce the amount of alcohol you drink; write them down, and then say them to yourself out loud.

1._____

2._____

3._____

Vitamins, Minerals, Herbs, and Spices

Vitamins and minerals...

"fat mind, fat body"

As we have discussed, a healthy diet consisting of a variety of grains, nuts, seeds, lean meats, oily fish, and fresh fruit and vegetables should allow you to meet all of your daily vitamin and mineral requirements. However, some of you may be more curious about what each of the different vitamins and minerals actually does for your health, the foods in which they can be found, and how much the recommended daily amount really is.

Q. Are you eating enough of the right foods to meet your requirements, and if not, what can you do to improve things?

A healthy diet is all about commitment; commitment to you and being the best you can be. If you recognise this, then you are well on the way towards achieving your goals.

Search online for an outline what the various vitamins and minerals do, their RDAs (Recommended Daily Amounts), and good dietary sources.

Remember, the key to a healthy diet is variety and getting a good mix of all the different sources mentioned.

"A little of what you fancy does you good."
- Marie Lloyd

Q. List three different vitamins or minerals found in whole grains?

Q. List three different vitamins or minerals found in your favourite fruit?

Salt

Too much salt or more accurately sodium, as table salt is sodium chloride, increases blood pressure and places extra stress on your heart, making a heart attack more likely. Most of the UK population eat too much salt, averaging around 9g a day compared to the recommended 6g. In order to lower your salt intake, the best advice is to avoid adding salt to the food you eat at the table. You can also use other spices in the foods you eat when cooking, for example, adding pepper increases the flavour of the salt you use so you are able to use less salt and still achieve the salty flavour you like. Avoiding processed ready meals and takeaways will also lower your salt intake as many of these products are high in salt to increase the shelf life.

Foods high in salt:

- Ready meals

- Bread

- Baked goods

- Takeaways

Drinking water, or other non-caffeinated drinks, in-between meals can help lower the effect of salt on your blood pressure. Increasing the potassium content of your diet has a similar effect.

Foods high in potassium:

- Low sodium salt

- Tomatoes

- Green leafy vegetables

- Bananas

- Seeds and nuts

When we exercise, we sweat, and salt is lost from the body through sweat along with other minerals. The salt lost must be replaced and if exercising at a moderate to high intensity for more than an hour, drinking a sports drink should replenish any salt and minerals lost through sweat. However, many people drink sports drinks when they are exercising less intensively and for shorter periods of time, and this can be counter- productive as the body uses the calories in the drink as fuel in preference to burning off fat to provide energy. If in doubt, only consume water.

The hidden danger of supplements...

If you are eating a balanced diet, you should be getting all of the essential nutrients you need. Whilst there may be some benefit to supplementing the diet with some products, most supplements have little evidence to support their often exaggerated health claims.

Also, supplements are often expensive; adding an extra expense to a family's budget – this represents the first hidden danger of supplements. The second hidden danger is the potential harmful effect on health. The fat-soluble vitamins, A, D, E, K, along with most minerals, build up in the body over time and can lead to toxicity. Scientists have recently uncovered some staggering evidence concerning the taking of mega dose supplements, meaning doses well above the RDA.

The CARET large scale trial of vitamin A intake's effect on cancer risk actually showed that the people taking mega dose vitamin A were more likely, not less likely to get lung cancer, as well as to die from it. In fact, the trial had to be finished early due to the increased risk. This finding also supported an earlier study that showed mega dose vitamin A and vitamin E supplementation increased cancer risk, adding weight to the concern that mega dose vitamins may actually do more harm than good.

With this understanding, taking mega dose vitamins is something you really should avoid, but if you are going to supplement your diet then use a supplement that is less than 100 per cent of your RDA to be on the safe side.

It might be tempting to rely on a pill to solve all your problems, rather than eating a healthy diet and exercising, but without changing your lifestyle; you will never keep the weight off for good. Also, there are many additional gains to be had through eating fruit and vegetables. As well as providing the vitamins and minerals your body needs, they also provide anti-oxidants, and when consumed in their natural form – in food rather than in a pill – they have a far greater effect; and popping healthy foods is much more enjoyable than popping a magic pill!

Smoking

Yes, you have probably heard it before but there is very little you can do that is worse for your health than smoking. On-going scientific research continues to back up the theory that smoking is not just bad for your own health, but for the health of everyone around you too.

There are over 4000 chemicals in cigarette smoke, many of which are toxic and carcinogenic (cancer causing). Smoking significantly increases the risk of cancer of the lung, throat, and pancreas as well as heart disease and stroke. Something many people may not know, however, is that smoking also hinders nutrient absorption in the body, affecting several areas of the digestive system. Consistent smoke inhalation, whether it be direct or passive inhalation, can lead to ulcers, liver disease, and Crohn's disease, all of which affect the absorption of nutrients from food. Smoking also impairs the liver's ability to process toxins, alcohol and other drugs, eventually leading to a damaged liver, further affecting the absorption of vital nutrients from the diet. As well as the abstract health effects, there are also many more negative effects that are deeply personal to you.

Q. Have you ever felt out of breath climbing the stairs, or running after the bus?

Q. How would it feel to be fitter, and healthier, able to keep up with that bus, or perhaps your partner or someone else in your life?

Q. What would your life be like if you could spend more time doing physical activities and being more active with your family and friends?

Quitting...

Remember to reinforce positive behaviours through the use of language. Start by reaffirming the belief that you don't need that cigarette. Tell yourself that going a day without smoking is a good thing; good for your health, your appearance, your friends, and your family.

Giving up smoking improves the taste of the food you eat as well as your overall experience of life.

Write down three things about your life that would improve if you gave up smoking.

1._____

Chapter Two

2._____

3._____

Tip: a close friend of mine shouted "six minutes" out load every time he wanted a cigarette. Why? He believed this was the average amount of time his life would be shortened by each time he lit up. It wasn't long before the embarrassment of saying "six minutes" in public was a strong enough motivator to stop saying it at all, and he stopped smoking.

If you need help to stop smoking or need to discuss your issues concerning alcohol, talk to your local health care department. They can offer support and advice, and will often have a national incentive scheme in place to assist you on your journey to a better you.

"fat mind, fat body"

Chapter Three

Exercise

"fat mind, fat body"

Why Exercise?

> *"Lack of activity destroys the good condition of every human being, while movement and methodical physical exercise save it and preserve it."*
>
> *- Plato*

A piece of research published in the American Journal of Clinical Nutrition by Kayman, Bruvold and Stern showed that 92 per cent of people who lost weight, and kept it off, exercised regularly. In the same study, only 34 per cent of those who lost weight but then put it back on again, exercised regularly. This is powerful evidence in support of the need to combine lifestyle, nutrition, and exercise.

The findings of the study can be explained by the fact that exercise increases your metabolic rate, the rate at which you burn off energy, not only during exercise but also at rest. With an appropriate exercise programme, your body will continue to burn a higher number of calories even after your exercise session, therefore continuing to burn off fat reserves. But, this is only part of the explanation, as it is also believed that exercise plays an important role in improving a person's psychological outlook. Specifically, exercise makes people feel good and may also lead to a lower risk of depression.

It has been scientifically proven that exercise stimulates an endorphin rush that elevates your general mood when exercising, generating an increased sense of wellbeing, and improving your overall self-image. Research has found that individuals who are intrinsically motivated to exercise, meaning they are focused on internal rewards such as how positive their improved fitness and weight loss is making them feel and the enjoyment of the exercise itself, are much more likely to stick with an exercise programme than individuals who are extrinsically motivated, meaning they are focused on external rewards such as a desire to change someone else's perception of them or to win a prize, or a bet. This highlights the importance of finding an exercise activity you enjoy, and want to take part in because of the way it makes you feel.

Emotion = energy and movement.

Think about it this way, the word "emotion" is defined by its break down. When broken down into two parts, the "e" relates to energy and the "motion" to the act of movement. Therefore, exercise or motion can have a direct impact on the way you feel, and on your energy levels. Right now, many people might say, "I feel terrible after exercise," but realistically, those who exercise as part of their day-to-day routine are proven to be happier emotionally. Using positive linguistics will allow you to focus on how much closer you are to achieving your goals, and how much better exercise makes you feel – not worse.

As you are now aware, weight gain occurs when you consume a greater number of calories than your body uses in its day-to-day tasks. Everything you eat contains calories and everything you do uses calories, from breathing and sleeping through to actually digesting the food you have eaten. Although reducing your daily intake of calories will help to reduce the amount of weight gained, and may aid in weight loss, the true key to losing weight lies in making your body burn, or use, more calories throughout the day to create the essential deficit. Cutting calories from your diet can be difficult and the more calories you need to cut, the more difficult it becomes. Exercising reduces the overall number of calories you need to trim from your diet. For example, through diet alone, you may need to cut 500 calories a day from the food you eat and this will obviously lead to significant changes in your eating habits. However, by combining diet and exercise, you can reduce the number of calories you need to cut to 250 in a day, using exercise to burn off the remaining 250 calories.

"fat mind, fat body"

As you can see, regular exercise is therefore a key element of effective weight loss. By using up your excess calories, it prevents your body from storing them as fat, and by contributing to a negative energy balance; exercise also aids you in your goal to lose weight. In addition, regular exercise helps to prevent many diseases, improves your overall health and fitness, and leads to a new, healthier, more energised you.

Q. How many hours a week do you exercise?

Q. What more would you do if you were physically fitter?

Fitness

If you don't currently exercise, you may find yourself becoming slightly out of breath when doing medial chores such as walking up flights of stairs or carrying lots of shopping bags. By changing your daily routine to include more time during the week for exercise, you promote the improvement of your cardiovascular system, which is the circulation of your blood from your heart around the body. This in turn will give you more energy to carry out your day-to-day tasks and help you achieve your goal of permanent weight loss. Improving your cardiovascular health also reduces your risk of heart disease, Type II diabetes, and a stroke.

> *"Those who think they have not time for bodily exercise will sooner or later have to find time for illness."*
> *- Edward Stanley*

By increasing your level of physical activity during the day, you can promote better sleep, falling asleep more quickly and achieving a deeper level of sleep, allowing you to wake feeling more refreshed and full of energy. Having a more efficient sleeping pattern also increases your ability to concentrate, improves your productivity, and boosts your mood. Improved rest will also make you more likely that you'll stick with your new lifestyle activities, such as eating better and exercising regularly. However, with that said, it's best to avoid exercising within two hours of going to bed as your improved energy and blood flow may, in this scenario, make it harder for you to drop off.

Getting Started

Making the initial push...

Begin by simply being more active in your daily life. With a little thought, you will find there are many different ways you can adapt your life to make it more active, for example:

- Getting off the bus a stop earlier and walking an extra ten minutes a day.

- Taking the stairs instead of the lift.

- Carrying items upstairs one at a time so that you make a return trip or two to the bottom instead of taking everything up with you in one trip.

Although only basic, these little adaptations can add up to an extra 10-60 minutes a day of otherwise avoided exercise. By increasing your energy expenditure, you will be taking the next step on the road to weight loss. Such changes should not be viewed as a one offs and should become routine habits, as the secret to achieving your goal is to make exercise a part of your daily life.

Think about one thing you can do right now to be more active tomorrow, make this a personal goal and dedicate yourself to

"fat mind, fat body"

achieving it.

To be more active, I will...

_____

_____

_____

_____

Remember, simply exercising for 20-30 minutes a day at a moderate intensity will soon improve your level of fitness and you will no longer have to worry about being out of breath when chasing that bus, or climbing those stairs.

What Do You Enjoy?

Everybody wants to be in shape and look good but why do some people manage to continue working out while others fall at the first hurdle? The simple answer is that people who work out on a continual basis enjoy it, and most importantly, understand the health benefits behind why they are working out.

As mentioned previously, having the right mindset is key. If you believe that exercise is boring, or pointless, and you can't see a reason for doing it, then you won't give it the attention needed in order to gain the associated benefits. By not positioning exercise highly enough on your list of priorities, you are creating another barrier between you and your weight loss goals. Reframing this situation and considering exercise as fun and important will make your brain consider all of the ways in which you can include the activities you enjoy within your exercise programme. For example,

Chapter Three

you may enjoy seeing friends, so how about meeting up with your friends to go swimming? The main thing to remember is that the best exercise you can do to lose weight is the exercise that you'll do!

The best form of exercise for you is any exercise you will do!

There is no point to doing exercises you hate or find boring, because the likelihood is you won't do them for very long or with any kind of commitment. It's essential that you enjoy the experience of losing weight.

Below are some popular forms of exercise that may give you some ideas; there's much more to exercise than joining a gym so perhaps there are a few you've not considered before?

Tip: Search online for a list of the number of calories each activity burns according to your body weight.

Rugby, Football, Netball, Hockey, Athletics, Running, Organised Classes, Boxing, Fast walking / Power walking, Jogging, Swimming, Dancing, Basketball, Jumping rope, Hiking, Rollerblading, Cross-country skiing, Tennis, Kickboxing, Push-ups, Stomach crunches, Lifting weights, Pull-ups, Biking, Martial Arts, Pilates, T'ai Chi, Yoga, Squash.

Q. What activities do you enjoy in your daily routine?

Q. What form of exercise can you carry out that includes the things you enjoy?

The list of potential activities is virtually endless, and some are going to attract your interest more than others, but who says that exercise has to be a task or chore? Surely there's an activity for each and every one of us to enjoy that actually helps us to burn calories at the same time. Maybe the thought of jogging is your worst nightmare and something you would never contemplate doing but something you do enjoy doing is walking around your local park. Begin there. Use the walk you enjoy as your starting point and then look for ways to increase the benefits of taking that walk. How about gradually increasing the distance, or perhaps decreasing the time it takes for to accomplish the walk? Make sure that whatever you decide to do is something you want to do, because if it's not, what's the likelihood that you are going to commit to the goal you have given yourself?

Even after broadening your horizons in terms of potential activities, there is always a small chance that exercise is going to be something you just really don't enjoy. If this is the case, finding an exercise you want to do is no longer an option so it becomes time to change your priorities. Losing weight through diet and exercise must now be reframed from a "want" to a "must" so, "I want to lose weight," or, "I need to lose weight" becomes, "I must lose weight, and without carrying out exercise, this just isn't going to happen." The fun factor is now no longer necessary and your mind will do whatever it can to ensure that you accomplish the things you must do. I promise you though, if you find something you enjoy doing, your journey will be a lot easier and most probably a lot quicker too.

No more excuses...

Every individual has commitments in their life that can be used as excuses to avoid carrying out things they know, inside, should be done. Be it work, kids, the shopping, cleaning, or having a night out, or in, with your girlfriend or boyfriend, procrastinating is only going to make the long-term pain of being overweight a lot harder to manage. Remember that the reason why you want to lose weight in the first place is to get rid of the pain you get from being overweight in your day-to-day life. The short-term pain of actually carrying out the plan you have structured to help lose the weight will always be far less than the pain you carried around with you because of the weight, otherwise you would never have started the programme in the first place.

We need to ensure that every commitment you have in your life is established and covered, so they can no longer be used as excuses to avoid exercise. If you have children to look after, ensure someone is there to look after them for you; if they need to be picked up from school, then perhaps make sure your time for exercise is whilst they are at school. If you're worried about encroaching on time spent with a partner, then why not take them with you on your morning jog, nothing is better that having someone to push and encourage you when you're feeling slightly lethargic. Or, if time is a problem, how about waking up an hour earlier than usual to make time for the gym or an exercise DVD at home. After all, if other people can make time for the gym and exercise, why can't you? Remember, we all share a 24-hour day, so it's up to you to choose what you do with those hours. A key and effective tip that I have seen used many times before is to have your trainers by the side of your bed with the socks sitting in them ready for you, and your exercise kit laid out ready to go. This way, when the alarm goes off for the first time slightly earlier than you're used to, there are no excuses. Remember, exercise is key to the weight loss you desire.

Organise your life around your exercise schedule and don't make excuses.

As all of us have different lifestyles, it must be said that these concepts are not going to work for everyone, but the ideas mentioned can help you to prepare for the many situations that life may throw your way, increasing the likelihood that you will achieve everything you want from your weight loss programme. By making sure you have every possible problem that may arise during your weight loss covered, you are eliminating excuses and increasing your chance for success.

Where...?

Q. Now that you have a fair idea of what you are going to include in your exercise program, where are you going to do it?

Where you decide to carry out the activities you desire depends wholly on the type of person you are and the lifestyle you live, as well as the exercise itself. The three most obvious choices are:

1. At home

2. Outdoors

3. Down the gym

Again, don't make excuses! Many of us use the excuse of not having a "local" gym to attend but most of us drive or have access to public transport so the number of gyms we could actually attend is probably much greater than we tell ourselves. Use an internet search engine or the Yellow Pages to look for gyms in your local area or close to your work. If you choose to exercise outdoors, a common excuse is the weather. With this in mind, a good plan is to choose a variety of activities that allow you to exercise in all weathers. For example, jogging around your local tree-lined park might be preferable to cycling out on the open road when it's raining. Mixing things up can also help to prevent boredom in your routine. Many people tell themselves they don't have enough space in their house to exercise, but in reality, how much space do you need for an exercise bike and a set of dumbbells? The answer of course is very little, and most of us have "wasted space" in our homes, space that is only being used because we haven't organised

Chapter Three

things effectively. Why not try reorganising your attic, cellar, garage, or spare room to take some of the clutter from your house and free the space for your exercise routine instead? Remember, even if you don't have space for an exercise bike, cross trainer, or treadmill you can still exercise in the comfort of your own home using exercise DVDs or a Wii (other brands of games consoles are of course available!)

At home...

Carrying out physical activity at home can be fantastic for people who do not wish to go out for a jog in the winter chill, or do not feel like going to a gym. A number of readily available, downloadable exercise programmes have been designed around exercising in the comfort of your own home. Of course, the cheapest and perhaps most obvious option is to put on one of your favourite CDs and dance around your living room. Doing the housework with gusto is another easy way to "work out" at home but there are a vast array of home fitness products available at affordable prices, such as skipping ropes, resistance bands, and abdominal machines. All you really need is enough space in your living room to get active without causing any accidental damage as getting the most from any activity means getting moderately out of breath.

Q. What exercises could you do at home?

Q. Which of these would you enjoy the most?

Outdoors...

The next option is to take advantage of the great outdoors. Taking a few extra brisk walks can easily provide massive health benefits through improved aerobic fitness, as long as you ensure that the

"fat mind, fat body"

intensity of your walk is high enough to increase your heart and breathing rate. The obvious next step from here would then be to go for a jog, run, or bike ride, all great options when the weather is nice and at no financial cost to you. If you have the option of joining a sports club, team sports are also a fantastic way to get involved in physical activity, providing not only an opportunity to meet new people but, after time, those people become a group of "team-mates" who depend on you to turn up. Team spirit can lead to feeling obliged to take part in the activities, but this in turn makes exercise a regular routine, leading to long-term weight loss.

Q. What are the advantages of carrying out exercises outdoors for you?

Q. What are the disadvantages?

Down the gym...

The last option, but often the first to spring to mind, is the gym. Your local gym will provide a number of exercise options, with everything from treadmills through to exercise bikes, or weight lifting through to organised classes, all providing different approaches to burning those calories. Using a variety of machines can reduce the tedium, and the programme options on each machine allow for variation in intensity in terms of speed and resistance so your workout can be tailored to suit your needs. However, one of the major benefits of attending a gym is that there's always a professional on hand to help you whenever you need it. They can offer advice on building a plan, or give guidance when you become stuck or feel that you are no longer improving, something you may not get when exercising in the comfort of your living room. If you prefer to work out as part of a group or need motivation from an external source, instructor-led classes (often included in memberships) are a great way to ensure you get the most out of your routine. Finally, many gyms also offer access to a swimming pool. Swimming provides a very low impact form of cardiovascular exercise, making it particularly useful for anyone carrying an injury or who happens to be frailer.

Q. What are the advantages of carrying out exercises at the gym for you?

Q. What are the disadvantages?

Q. Where could you see yourself carrying out your weekly exercises?

When, How Long, and How Often?

The answer to the question of "how long" depends on your own individual goal and what it is you wish to achieve. The general recommendation for overall cardiovascular fitness in relation to weight loss is to exercise three to five times a week, with each session lasting between 30 to 60 minutes. However, this is obviously just a guideline, and if you were to carry out a regular 60 minute session, you may not need to do as many sessions in a week as you would if you were to carry out a regular 30 minute session. Exercise is essentially a long-term routine that you should make a part of your life for the foreseeable future. It is not just a short-term answer. The amount of time you choose to allocate to exercise is entirely down to you. Bear in mind that you can allocate the time devoted to each exercise session differently, for example, you may have enough time to work out for an hour on a Saturday but only enough time to exercise for 30 minutes on week days.

The current Department for Health guidelines state that for improvements in health, and to begin to lose weight, you should exercise for around two and a half hours each week at a moderate intensity, or one and quarter hours at a high intensity. This recommendation can be split into as many sessions as you like. For example, you may choose to do two fifteen minute workouts a day for five days each week, or you may choose to do two one hour workouts and one half hour workout in a week, the choice is yours and the benefits remain the same. By using a combination of the above recommendations, and the knowledge provided by working out your energy balance and the fact that it takes around 3500 calories to burn a pound of fat, you can now decide on and create a routine that is tailored to your own personal needs and goals.

Q. How many sessions a week will you fit into your lifestyle?

It is important to start slowly, even if you are someone who exercised regularly in the past, as doing too much too soon can lead to overtiredness and potentially injury. Many people who used to exercise in the past, start off at the same pace they left off at, only to discover that their body has changed and is not as fit and efficient as it once was. If you have been inactive for some time, don't throw on your trainers with the intention of going on a ten mile run straight away.

If a 30-minute session seems too much to start off with, perhaps start with a 10-minute routine for the first week or two to begin building fitness or to get back into the swing of things. You can then begin to slowly increase the length of your routine and the intensity at which you exercise. Remember that you are not only there to lose weight but to enjoy the journey, therefore you don't want to push yourself so hard that you are going to hate it and not want to do it again. Research indicates that people who start off exercising at too high an intensity have a very high dropout rate, whereas those who begin at a lower intensity and work their way up as their fitness improves tend to continue on their exercise programme for longer.

Chapter Three

The only person who will truly know when you are tired or how much exercise is right for you is you. Be truthful and ensure that you work at a level that is slightly out of your comfort zone as it's important to challenge your body when you exercise. Listen to your body; if your muscles or joints start to hurt, or your breathing becomes difficult or uncomfortable, you need to slow down. Remember that exercising for weight loss is a marathon and not a sprint. You need to be fit enough for your next workout, and the next.

This is going to be a long-term achievement and it's not going to happen overnight.

As mentioned earlier, everyone is an individual with their own goals and ways of achieving them, but, as a rule of thumb, for every mile you walk or run, around 100 calories are burnt – give or take. Another way of looking at it is that for every half hour of relatively high intensity activity, around 300 calories are burnt, depending on your weight and level of activity. By increasing your level of activity by 300 calories a day and continuing to eat the same amount, you will achieve a 1500 calorie reduction in just one week – all from just 30 minutes of exercise a day. When you add exercise to your new nutrition plan, the calorie deficit you create will inevitably lead to weight loss, and not only will you lose weight, you will also gain more energy.

How Much is This Going to Cost Me?

It's a common misconception that exercising and getting in shape is going to cost a lot of money. This is true if you choose to pay for gym membership, a personal trainer, specialist equipment... and the list goes on. But, to be honest we could make a long list of unessential and exceptionally expensive excuses as to why we are going to put off doing the exercise we need to do. At the end of the day, all you really need is a pair of comfortable trainers and the open road, and you have a perfect exercise programme.

With that said, a personal trainer can be invaluable. Along with their mountain of exercise knowledge, they also provide a positive driving force, making it possible for you to work out at your optimum by pushing you beyond your comfort zone, but also knowing just where and when to stop. If you can't afford a personal trainer and need to know the answer to an exercise question, why not ask the internet? Google has the answer to many a question you may need answering, and the probability is that somebody has already asked it, and therefore somebody may already have answered it. However, choose your sources carefully. Similarly, if you can't afford a personal trainer but want that extra level of motivation, why not exercise with a friend who also wants to get in shape. What's stopping you arranging to meet a friend to go for a regular jog three times a week? Your friend can offer you the support structure you need to stick with your plan at no extra cost, and they don't even need to be exercising themselves to be able to give you encouragement and a push you when you need it.

Perhaps you do want to sign up to a gym, but can't quite justify the cost to yourself. The bottom line is that a gym membership is only worth as much as you are going to use it. The more you visit the gym per month, the cheaper your average visit becomes, but if you subscribe to a membership and then never go, it's costing you a lot. Why not take the first step now and find out how much it costs to see whether it is a feasible option?

Q. How much is it to sign up to your local gym?

Q. How many times will you use it a month?

Q. Dividing your overall monthly cost by how often you are going to use it, how much is each session going to cost you?

Q. What can you stop buying in your life to fund this?

Q. How is going to the gym worth it to you?

If cost is not a problem, consider getting some sort of coach or mentor in your life. They are professionals who work from day-to-day at specifically improving the quality of other people's lives, and are very good at it. Health coaches work hand-in-hand with you to assist you in achieving your personal wellness goals. They can directly help you change and adapt your lifestyle and habits to help you become the person you've always wanted to be.

It all narrows down to how much money you are willing to put forward into investing in your human capital, improving your way of life. You can partake in physical activity at any cost that suits you, be it for little or nothing up to costing a lot, it all comes down to you as an individual. Cost does not need to be an excuse, as there doesn't have to be any. All that said, there are a few pointers that can be used in your everyday life to help you save a little.

Instead of consulting an expensive personal trainer on a one-to-one level, why not purchase a fitness DVD at a minimal cost. Choose one that has been produced by a personal trainer or someone who has already cut the weight, and it becomes the most financially beneficial way of getting a coach into your living room. The best thing about it is that you can use it over and over again.

Gyms also often give away free trials such as a free week, or 10 free sessions. If you simply multiply the number of free days by the number of gyms around your local area, you'll find that you may gain weeks of gym membership at no cost to you whatsoever.

Exercise Programmes

How can an exercise programme help me...?

Using an exercise programme can be a great way of keeping track of what you have to do on a certain day and what you have done over the past few days, weeks and months. Nothing is better than seeing an improvement in strength, stamina, and flexibility, especially when you have it written in black and white in front of you. When you begin to see results, it will drive you to work harder on a more regular basis. Reaping the rewards is the best part of achieving anything in life. It must be warned however that when you start to exercise and see results, it can very quickly become addictive.

Whether designing your fitness programme yourself or getting a professional to help you, it is always key to remember your goals, as they are the reasons why you are doing what you are doing. To ensure you reach your goal, make sure to include exercises that you are going to enjoy, ones that you like. It's also important that your programme doesn't start too intensely, but is forever progressing and getting more difficult. If you always train at the same level, you will never improve, so make sure your programme is constantly getting a little more challenging and mix things up.

Allow yourself time to recover, as recovery time is key to keeping your body in a position to train at its optimum in the following session. After a particularly heavy training session, make sure you get lots of sleep, and train on consecutive days rather than two days in a row, in order to allow time for your muscles to recover. Keep listening to your body as your muscles are a good indicator of when you're doing too much – they're going to let you know. If you become sore, it's okay to take an extra day off, as working too hard is not an enjoyable way to exercise. Over time, you will find that your body adapts to the activity you are doing and those aches and pains become less common between exercise sessions.

Chapter Three

The best place to get an exercise programme is from a gym. Many gyms offer a free consultation on signing up with them, along with a monthly or bimonthly review to see how you are doing relative to your goals and to put appropriate changes in place. Other than this, it is possible to gather enough information from books or the Internet to build your own personalised exercise plan. If you do decide to design your own plan, make sure you put it on paper, or create a dedicated file on your computer, as a written plan will help you stay on track and avoid missing out important elements of your programme. You could also ask a professional to have a look over it for you to check that it's accurate and that it contains appropriate exercises to help you attain your goals.

Measure your progress...

When putting together an exercise programme, the first question you may be asked, or need to ask yourself is, "What's your current fitness level?" You probably have some idea of how fit you are but by measuring your fitness in a consistent manner, you will have a benchmark you can use in the future to compare results and gauge your progress. There are a number of methods you can use depending on the specific area of fitness you are looking to improve. The key is to ensure that the method you use is measurable and repeatable, so that you can use exactly the same method to re-test in the future.

For example, let's say you're going to measure your pulse before and after doing 30 minutes of exercise. To be able to measure and gauge your progress accurately, you will need to record the exact exercises being used along with the duration and intensity so that in repeat tests, you are able to create exactly the same conditions. Small changes in the conditions such as the weather or the time of day can also affect your results. If the first test was carried out in cold weather at lunchtime and the follow-up test was carried out on a hot day in the evening after work, the changes in environment will need to be taken into consideration. There are many simple ways to test your fitness levels, for example:

- How many press-ups you can do in a minute?

- How quickly can you run a mile?

- How many circuits of the circular route in your local park can you walk in a specified time?

- What's your resting pulse rate 10 minutes after completing a specified exercise?

Aim to monitor your progress at regular intervals throughout your programme. Plan to re-test your fitness at appropriate intervals, perhaps every five to six weeks or so. By repeating your original benchmark test, you can see just how much you have improved, and the sense of achievement this creates provides a motivational boost to keep going. If you find you have not improved, you now have an opportunity to analyse your results and use the feedback as a way to make positive adjustments that will get your programme back on track.

The more varied you can make your programme; the less potential there is for you to become bored. Use variety to make every training day feel like a new start rather than the same old routine time and time again. Remember, the exercise you enjoy is the best exercise for you, but too much of a good thing can be bad for you too, so mix it up.

The Warm Up

Chapter Three

Although frequently overlooked, the warm up is an essential part of your programme if you are to give your body the best chance to perform at its optimum. Contrary to popular opinion, a warm up routine should not involve static stretches such as reaching down to touch your toes, but should involve dynamic stretches and exercises. Dynamic exercises gently prepare your muscles for the activity ahead by taking your body through the range of movements involved in the exercise ahead at a lower intensity, without resistance or weight other than bodyweight. After a general warm up, exercises such as lunges and squats continue to stretch the muscles, improve the flow of blood, and reduce the potential for injury when the intensity increases. Warm muscles are more elastic than cold muscles, therefore less prone to injury, so with this in mind, static stretches such as toe touching or doing the splits can actually increase the potential for injury by overstretching the muscles before they are warm. However, static stretches can be used as part of your programme on a separate day dedicated to improving your flexibility, or at the end of an exercise session as part of your warm down.

High Intensity Interval Training

One type of training that deserves a special mention in relation to developing your exercise programme is high intensity interval training, also known as HIIT. This style of training involves working out at a high intensity, 80 per cent of your maximum heart rate or a level where talking is no longer possible, for a short period of time and then exercising at a moderate intensity for another period. The ratio of these periods is usually one to one, one to two, or one to three. For example, you could exercise on an exercise bike for three minutes at a moderate intensity followed by one, two, or three minutes at a high intensity, and then repeat for an allocated total period of time. HIIT works your heart harder than other routines and leads to a boost in your fat metabolism, so you will continue to burn off more calories even when you're not exercising. It's a training method that can be worked into just about any training programme. For example, if you are swimming you could sprint swim every third lap, maintaining a moderate intensity on the other laps. This is also a useful way of mixing up your routine and breaking down an exercise period so that time seems to pass faster, making it more likely that you'll stick to your programme in the long run.

Cardiovascular Training

Cardiovascular exercises are the best type of training exercises to improve the efficiency of your heart, lungs, and the circulatory system, as well as aiding your weight loss. Jogging, running, and cycling are all well-known examples of cardiovascular exercises that can help you to burn off more calories. But many other sports and activities such as football, martial arts, and playing Frisbee in the park also have a strong cardiovascular component to them. By boosting your cardiovascular system, you will gain a wealth of health benefits in addition to improving your overall fitness. Aim to train your cardiovascular system at least three times per week, but in order to lose weight and then keep it off, you also need to consider building resistance exercises into your routine.

Resistance Training

Resistance exercises are exercises that place an additional strain on your body and so to some extent all exercises have a resistance component. However, exercises such as weight training, yoga, and pilates all place an additional strain on your body, helping to promote muscle tone and growth, and thereby boosting your metabolism. Weight training is an especially effective form of resistance training but thoughts of training with weights may conjure up images of muscle-bound body builders huffing away down the gym! However, many different types of people use weight training as part of their exercise regime and as it boosts fat metabolism, it is often seen as the exercise secret to permanent weight loss. It's not necessary to lift heavy weights; the weights you use only need to be heavy enough to provide an appropriate challenge for your body. Correct posture and exercise technique is extremely important when using weights so ask a professional, fellow gym member or friend with weights experience to help you so that injury can be avoided. It's also possible to use the Internet to research correct exercise technique with many reputable websites providing video demonstrations and step-by-step instructions.

A good rule of thumb when using weights is the **two second up and two second down technique.**

• Take your time, allowing two seconds to lift the weight to the end point

• Maintain tension in the muscle and avoiding jerking movements

• Take another two seconds to lower the weight to the start point

• Again, maintain tension in the muscle, squeezing the working muscle at the end of the lift

In resistance training, each exercise is broken down into sets and each set is broken down into repetitions. As a general guide to finding the correct weight for you, aim to use a weight that allows you to perform no more than 15 repetitions per set, for the total number of sets. By your final set, achieving all 15 repetitions should be a physical impossibility, perhaps managing to complete 10 to 12 repetitions before reaching failure, meaning you are unable to complete another lift. An example might be as follows:

Leg Press (fixed weight machine)

Set 1 = 12 to 15 repetitions

Short rest of up to 1 minute

Set 2 = 12 to 15 repetitions

Short rest of up to 1 minute

Set 3 = 12 to 15 repetitions (or repetitions to failure)

For optimum health benefits, you should aim to use resistance training at least twice per week with at least one day of training without weights in-between sessions. Non-weight training days can be cardiovascular training days or rest days.

The Warm Down

A warm down is essentially a warm up in reverse. Just as a warm up gently prepares your body for exercise by warming up the muscles, a warm down allows your muscles to cool down gently which helps to minimise the potential for soreness after exercise. Low intensity aerobic exercises such as a slow jog or brisk walk (or jogging or marching on the spot) allow your heart rate to slow down while keeping the blood flowing around your muscles. This helps to shake the build up of lactic acid out of your muscles, as it's lactic acid that gives your muscles that fuzzy, heavy feeling during and then after exercise. After lowering your heart rate, but while your muscles are still warm, warm down stretches help to return muscles that may have shortened during exercise to their normal length. This is important as shortened muscles are responsible for that tight, uncomfortable feeling you may have experienced after exercise, and tight, inflexible muscles are much more prone to injury. Skipping the warm down at the end of a session may lead to suffering an injury in your next session.

Sample Routines

Beginner...

After two to three weeks of relatively gentle activity aimed at building up exercise tolerance, a beginner's exercise regime may look something like this:

Monday: Warm up, cardio 20-30 minutes, followed by a warm down.

You could choose from the following cardio workouts: walking, cycling, running – in the gym or outdoors, or alternatively, star jumps, bunny hops, and jogging on the spot if at home.

Tuesday: Warm up, total body strength and core training 20-30 minutes, followed by a warm down.

For example, weight training using full body exercises such as squats, overhead raises, bench press, and dead-lift, or if outdoors, bodyweight exercises such as chin ups, crunches, and press ups.

Wednesday: Rest day or gentle stretching such as relaxation yoga.

Thursday: Repeat Monday's cardio regime, mixing it up as desired.

Friday: Repeat Tuesday's resistance training routine, mixing it up as desired.

"fat mind, fat body"

Saturday: Repeat the cardio routine with variations as desired.

Sunday: Rest day.

Tip: Resistance-training activities can be combined with cardio training if you want to exercise on fewer days.

This routine would typically be carried out for around six weeks then it would be changed, for example, resistance could be increased. By mixing up your exercise selections, you keep your routine interesting and shake your body up, preventing it from getting too used to the exercises you are doing. Remember, your body will always try to find the most efficient way of doing an exercise and the weight loss effect of a particular exercise will diminish over time as it adapts to the challenge. It takes new, progressive challenges to keep getting the maximum benefit from your exercise sessions. However, avoid any temptation to exercise for more than two hours in a day, as this will increase the amount of time it takes your muscles to recover.

Intermediate...

An intermediate's regime – someone who has been exercising regularly for around six months – may look a little like this:

Monday: Warm up, cardio 30-60 minutes, followed by a warm down.

You may wish to try incorporating high intensity interval training into your workout. See the beginner's routine for example exercises.

Tuesday: Warm up, total body strength and core training 30-60 minutes, followed by a warm down.

You may now want to vary the full body exercises listed in the beginner's routine. Alternatively you may want to try including isolation exercises aimed at toning up specific muscle groups such as bicep curls, triceps kickbacks, and dumbbell fly's. When doing isolation exercises, target upper body and lower body on different days.

Wednesday: Rest day or gentle stretching such as relaxation yoga.

Thursday: Repeat Monday's cardio regime, mixing it up as desired.

Friday: Repeat Tuesday's resistance training routine, but if using isolation exercises, target the areas of your body not exercised on Tuesday. Mix up the exercises up as desired.

Saturday: Repeat the cardio routine as desired.

Sunday: Rest day.

Tip: Remember, weight training and cardio sessions can be combined for a longer workout as desired. When doing isolation exercises, use a maximum of four different exercises per targeted muscle group.

Advanced...

An advanced routine, for someone who has been exercising regularly for a year or more, may look like this:

Monday: Warm up, cardio 40-60 minutes, followed by a warm down.

See the example exercises listed above. By now you should be using high intensity interval training in your cardio workouts.

Tuesday: Warm up, target body section strength training 30-60 minutes, followed by a warm down.

Your resistance training routine should now be split up into at least three target body sections, for example, arms and chest, abdominals, and lower body.

Wednesday: Rest day or gentle stretching such as relaxation yoga.

Thursday: Repeat Monday's cardio regime, mixing it up as desired, followed by target body section resistance training for around 30 minutes.

Friday: Repeat Tuesday's resistance training session but this time target a different section of your body, mixing the exercises up as desired. This routine should be around 30-60 minutes.

Saturday: Repeat the cardio routine as desired.

Sunday: Rest day.

Tip: Remember, your routine can be as simple or as complicated as you want it to be, and the most important activity for you to do is any activity that you will do.

You don't have to exercise yourself into the ground or spend forever in the gym in order to mix things up a little and create new challenges. Many of the ideas presented above can be built into the sports and hobbies you enjoy. For example, interval training can be built into football practise; indeed many coaches already use intervals regularly in training. Or, when playing squash with a friend, you can include high intensity periods of play where you really push each other hard, mixed with less intense periods of play. When running or jogging, you can vary the intensity by jogging backwards or side-skipping for a period, and hill work or speed drills are a great way to add a new challenge to interval training. There are many ways you can build both resistance and intensity into the exercises and sports you do.

Other ways of mixing up an exercise routine...

When you reach an intermediate or advanced level of training, some other techniques that may be useful in terms of mixing up your routine include the following:

Pyramiding

Pyramiding is a method of increasing intensity and adding interest in weight training. It involves starting off at a lower weight or resistance than you can tolerate – around 60 per cent of the weight you could feasibly lift or move once – for the first set, and then gradually increasing the weight in each of the following sets until your muscles reach failure. The number of repetitions in each set is normally 4-15 with the number of reps decreasing as the weight increases. It is common to increase the resistance by 10 per cent of your maximum lift each set, and the tip of the pyramid is normally achieved when lifting 80 to 90 per cent of your maximum lift for around four repetitions. After this, the weight is decreased by the same amount it was increased on consecutive sets until back to the start, although this time you will manage fewer repetitions at each weight than before.

Supersets

Supersets can be combined into any weight training or resistance programme to increase intensity, improve muscle tone, and shock the body into shedding those unwanted pounds. In simple terms, supersets are sets done back to back with no rest in-between. This can be done to target different body parts one after the other. For example, you may wish to do press-ups to failure followed by sit-ups with no rest in-between, or you may wish just to do all the sets of one exercise with no gap for a breather.

Circuit training

Circuit training describes itself in that it is simply training in a circuit. Whatever type of training you are doing, cardio or resistance, you perform the various exercises as a circuit, or lap, moving from exercise to exercise until one complete circuit is finished before pausing for breath. For example, you could run for 15 minutes, followed by skipping or jogging on the spot for five minutes, then do press-ups to failure before pausing to take a brief breather before repeating the circuit.

Am I too old?

Older age groups and the frail...

You are never too old to lose weight. It's true that your body changes and high impact activities such as running may no longer be an option but don't worry, it's still possible to cut the pounds. Low impact activities such as walking, swimming, or using elliptical trainers can help you to increase the number of calories you burn each day. Exercising your joints in any form of low impact activity will improve your circulation and make your day-to-day life easier.

Wouldn't you like to walk more easily? If you can manage even a small amount of exercise on a daily basis, whether it's going for a walk or going ballroom dancing, you can reduce the risk of many of the diseases common in later life. Just two to three minutes of exercise at a high intensity each day can reduce your risk of developing Type II diabetes and improve insulin sensitivity. Remember, intensity is personal to you; what is high intensity for one person is not necessarily high intensity for the next, so always do what you can manage.

There are a variety of group exercises classes designed specifically for older exercisers, with everything from aqua-aerobics through to "chair-obics" for those who are less mobile. Exercising in a group can add to the fun and provide an added source of motivation and support. It's important not to put yourself at risk as you exercise so exercising with a friend is advisable, or at the very least, exercise with a phone within easy reach. Exercising with younger relatives is another good way to help boost your metabolism and improve your circulation, balance, and joint health. Perhaps you have a nephew, or grandchild who has one of the new consoles with inbuilt motion sensors? Playing games together is a great way to turn exercise into a fun, family event.

Am I too young?

Exercise and children...

Many children are now overweight, if not obese, and this number is growing all the time. Exercise in childhood can help to prevent the onset of weight related conditions such as heart disease, Type II diabetes, and bone and joint problems in later life. It can also improve a child's emotional health, helping to generate a positive

"fat mind, fat body"

self-image and boost self-confidence. Resistance training using weights is not advised in younger age groups when the body is still growing, and even in teenage years should only be done as part of an instructor-led exercise class. However, if you have a child with weight concerns, begin by finding out what interests them. Traditional sports may not motivate them to exercise but other activities such as dancing, skateboarding, or roller-skating may spark their interest, and getting them involved in a sport or hobby they will enjoy is the best way to encourage weight loss.

Maybe you could do a sport or activity as a family, tai chi or a more gentle martial art for example? By encouraging your children to exercise, you will be changing their lives for the better. Avoid directly confronting your child about their weight, as this will often only add to the negative feelings they may have about themselves. Instead, encourage and reward positive behaviour, for example, allowing them to stay up later on the days they have exercised, even when it's as simple as playing football with their friends in the park. Currently, many girls in particular stop exercising around puberty due to body issues and poor self-image, so it's important to bear this in mind and offer support during this often-difficult period.

Weight Loss Exercises For the Mind

As well as weight loss exercises for the body, there are a variety of weight loss exercises for the mind that can help you on your journey to being the you that you want to be.

Question Your Feelings

Start by thinking about everything you associate with those fatty treats – pleasure, excitement, the mouth watering, succulence of the melting flavours? Now think about the feelings you believe those dirty, fatty, non-nutritional foods will bring – happiness, relief, power, or perhaps control? Now think about whether those feelings are actually true, or whether it's your mind playing tricks on you.

The truth, if you haven't already guessed, is that your body doesn't actually crave those disgusting non-essential foods, but your mind wants them because of the psychological feelings you have associated with them. By taking a critical overview of this, perhaps by getting a third party perspective, you'll be able to see clearly that dieting on its own won't change those feelings nor will it allow you to make the long-term changes you desire. These "quick fixes" will only suppress those feelings and will usually create a sense of guilt and resentment. Using the visualisation within the hypnosis audios, you will be able to delete those feelings towards un-supporting foods and transfer them to the nutritionally rich foods you should desire.

Word Changes

Over the coming days, make a conscious choice to remove these words from your vocabulary. These words being those that most likely offer you acceptance and closure; acceptance that being overweight is fine. The aim is to remove these words to ensure that weight gain is not acceptable; you do not accept being overweight as being fine and you do not want to be fat or have ownership over those few extra pounds.

Think about it like this, how often do you not want something and yet you keep it? Rarely! You wouldn't keep rubbish in your kitchen for months on end without getting rid of it would you? You would put it out in the street to be collected on a weekly basis and remove it, simply because you no longer need it and don't want it.

The same attitude must be had with weight loss and the toxins held within the fatty deposits in your body.

Words to change or delete until your habits are properly formed...

Try - you'll never succeed when you "try" to complete something. Change try to will. Saying "I will" adds the natural assumption that you will complete it without any doubt. Think about it for a second, how many times have you ever completed something when you "tried" to do it?

Am/Mine/My – ownership is something that all of us like to have, however, ownership of unnecessary weight is something you need to let go. Be careful when referring to "your" weight. Start to talk in the past context. Talk about your weight as something you had in the past and not in the present, simply doing this will add disassociation to your views on weight. "I was big but I am getting thinner" or, "I used to be fat but I am not anymore."

Can't – I remember using the word "can't" during my army basic training; my training corporal at the time seemed to enjoy lecturing me on the use and power of that incantation. He said, "Can't means cannot. Cannot means can but you're not going to; not doing what I am asking means disobeying a direct order!" Can't is one of the most powerful incantations commonly used every day. Start to change the sentence structure when normally using this word. Change, "I can't do this!" to "how can I do this?" When you say you can't have something, what do you naturally want? Substituting this situation with reason will often deflect the feelings of loss, for example, "I can't have a chocolate bar" reframed to, "I can have a mixed fruit snack instead of a chocolate bar because it's nutritionally more beneficial and supports my wellbeing." Notice the changes on a neurological level within your body.

Won't – won't is the same as can't, so you should follow the routines already outlined above.

Loss – loss is associated with all of the most emotional events in our life; the loss of a loved one, the loss of a job, or the loss of an opportunity can all trigger negative feelings. Avoid where possible using the word "loss", for example, using the term weight loss. It isn't lost, but no longer needed.

Although there are many more, the above are the ones that will mostly likely be noticed and used most frequently. If you need to, keep a note in your purse or wallet, making it visible every time you open it, as a way of reminding yourself of these word changes.

The Art of Replacement

If you make a space within anything there will always be a sense that something is missing, just as if you take a picture off a wall that has been there for many years, you will notice it, and it will often create a sense that something is missing. This of course is the body's natural ability to notice change; unfortunately this sense of emptiness will often cause us to fill it in order to feel complete.

When changing your diet and nutritional intake, it is essential that you substitute everything you do. If you take out a regular fatty snack and fail to replace it, your body will crave the loss of that routine event. To add to this, when making such drastic changes to your lifestyle it's important to avoid using the "can't" word as in this context, it often creates negative wants and desires.

When you say, "I can't have this," your mind works out all of the reasons why you should have this.

"fat mind, fat body"

Remember, your mind only focuses on the positives, and will often read "I can have this." Replace everything you have been accustomed to, and make small changes. Drastic changes will only recoil you back into that state of loss, which isn't productive. Remember that you are missing out on more by being overweight than through being healthy. If you need to, just replace two things per day to keep it simple and progressive.

Change your attention to the new, thinner you...

As mentioned on several occasions within this book, you become what you think about the most. In the past you were big because that's what you focused on, now, more than likely, you are focused on becoming a healthier, vibrant, more confident person than you currently are. What is important, is that you keep this focus throughout the rest of your life.

Doing this initially may seem like a bit of challenge, however, once programmed in and habitual, this will form part of your daily life without conscious thought. To get started, think yourself thin. Although this is a fairly "airy fairy" statement, it's scientifically proven that the more you use your mind to create a belief structure aimed at a healthy living, the more you'll bring about those opportunities that allow this to happen. Think about it this way, if you think "fat" you may notice all of the things that support being fat, such as fatty foods, lack of exercise, and the list goes on. Along with this you will label those situations, events, or opportunities as negative. If however you change your thinking and focus towards a "thin" body, you'll notice all of the things that support this.

The truth is that in the past your focus and attention was drawn to all of the reasons why you were overweight with any negative event simply highlighting this, causing a defensive attitude to protect yourself from harm. Therefore, over the next few days, I would like you to notice all of the positive healthy things that will support you in obtaining the lifestyle you wish. You do not have to partake in any change just yet, just notice. If you need to, keep a list of all of the things that will remind you to think thin.

Old Wives Tales and Frequently Asked Questions

Q. Surely to reduce your calorie intake, it is a good idea to stop eating regular meals, or reduce the amount of meals you eat in a day, because if you stop eating regular meals you won't eat as much, right?

A. Wrong! You should aim to achieve the calorie deficit necessary for weight loss through no more than a one to one ratio between calories burnt in exercise and dietary restriction. That is, no more than 50 per cent of the calorie reduction needed for weight loss should be achieved through diet, and your total calorie deficit should not exceed 1000 calories. Any more than this and you risk affecting your metabolism and reducing the number of calories you burn at rest and throughout the day. The body needs a certain amount of calories each day to function properly. Each one of us is an individual. We each must eat an amount of food that meets our individual requirements and as we won't all carry out the same amount of physical activity and we aren't all the same body weight, or composition, this amount is different for each of us.

The key to successful weight loss and calorie restriction is to keep a track of your intake and expenditure. If you are an active person, you will burn more calories than someone who is less active. Too few calories and your body begins to shut down; it receives the message that for whatever reason, there is going to be a famine and your body enters "starvation" mode. When this happens, the food you do eat is more likely to be stored as fat, as the body's metabolism slows down, leaving you feeling tired, lethargic, and sluggish.

Q. Why not just crash diet, surely that would be easier?

A. No. If you have come to the conclusion that by crash dieting, you will be able to cut the kilos really quickly at no harm to yourself at all, you are wrong. This is definitely not the case. When a person begins to lose weight, the first place it starts to become noticeable is in the face, and then the weight slowly comes off the lower segments of your body. Basically, your body lays down fat preferentially in certain areas and these areas are the last to become visibly reduced. If you are intending to lose weight in a more specific place, such as your thighs or stomach, then crash dieting will definitely not work. Yes, people will notice a difference in your appearance, but for all the wrong reasons. Your face will begin to look slightly saggy and your skin will lose its tension, along with a reduction in chest size and looseness around the upper arms. The reason for this is that you are starving your body of all the essential vitamins and minerals it needs to maintain its healthy look.

It is better to reduce your intake of calories by watching what you eat rather than by heavily slashing calorie intake. This will ensure that you are still getting all of the essential vitamins, minerals, and other nutrients you need, allowing your body to maintain itself to the standard that you desire and with the overall look you want. If you starve your body, your metabolism will slow down and therefore burn food more slowly. If you dehydrate it, it will hold the water it has, as it is scared it won't gain any more for a while, leading to water retention. Both of the above situations are awful if weight loss is your desired outcome. Crash diets are to be avoided at all costs.

Q. My fat is because I have a slow metabolism, isn't it?

Chapter Three

A. In two words, probably no. Some people do have conditions that make them more likely to gain weight, an under-active thyroid gland being the primary culprit, but this represents a tiny proportion of the population and if you suspect you have an under active thyroid, you really should speak to your doctor. For most people trying to lose weight, this is not the case. Whilst it is true that people have different speeds of metabolism and therefore some people can break down their food quicker than others, it is also true that you can control the speed of your metabolism to some extent. If you only eat one meal a day, your metabolism is going to be slower than those who eat three to four regularly spaced and smaller sized meals a day, as their metabolism will constantly be stimulated by the process of digesting the food they eat. The more fat you burn, the more pounds, and therefore inches, you will lose, this is a fact. The more regular your eating pattern, the quicker your metabolism; the quicker your metabolism, the quicker you will lose weight. Exercise also stimulates your metabolism, as does drinking, so if you have regular glasses of water and make exercise a part of your life, you should have no problems with a sluggish metabolism.

Q. If I don't eat my crusts, I'll never get hairs on my chest, will I?

A. When I was younger, my mother always told me that if I didn't eat every part of my bread, I would never get hairs on my chest. This is something she'd tell me one week and then the following week she'd tell me that if I didn't eat every part of my bread, my hair would never curl. Personally, I never wanted either, but that's neither here nor there, the question is, is that really true?

Although eating a load of bread perhaps isn't the best thing to do when you have decided that you want to lose weight, some research shows that the crust of a piece of bread actually contains eight

"fat mind, fat body"

times as many antioxidants as any other part of the bread. So, if you have the option, always eat the crust!

Q. If I eat an apple a day, will the doctor really stay away?

A. Many doctors have disagreed with the saying that eating an apple a day will keep the doctor away. Instead, they have come to the general consensus that the only way you are going to keep them away is by throwing the apple at them. Researchers have announced that as apples contain a high level of polyphenols, which work as antioxidants, they can help reduce the risk of both breast and colon cancer, with other research suggesting that it may also help you in avoiding Alzheimer's disease. So, although it won't keep the doctor at bay forever or for everything, it may keep him away a little longer due to your efficiently balanced diet.

Q. I have always finished every carrot I am given yet still go bump in the night. Can they really help me see in the dark?

A. Although a nice concept, it has been proven that someone who already has a balanced diet will not gain improved eyesight, during the day or night, from eating more carrots. A diet that already holds sufficient Vitamin A, iron, and pro vitamins, which are vital for the health of your eyes, will mean that an individual's sight will be at its optimum.

There are two sources of vitamin A. Carotenoids, found in carrots, are not as good a source as the retinol found in apples and liver, but can still contribute to your vitamin A requirements, especially if you are running at a deficiency. If you have vitamin A deficiency, you are at risk of a condition known as night blindness where your eyes struggle to adapt to changes in light. This is due to the large amounts of retinol involved in making the retina, a key part of your eye. This is probably the source of this old wives tale.

Chapter Three

Q. Is Popeye a suitable person to model, and do his dietary tactics of spinach really make him that strong?

A. Because of Popeye, eating spinach has been renowned for increasing your strength, but is this really true? Spinach holds a lot of antioxidants, helping to prevent cancer later on in life, and also has very few calories, meaning that you can eat a lot of it without having to worry too much about the effect on your waistline. It is also a rich source of fibre and vitamin C, and is a good source of iron for vegetarians. Iron is essential for transporting oxygen from the lungs to the working muscles, and for storing the oxygen in the muscles, although there is only so much iron that the body needs and therefore only so much that is able to be absorbed. The rest is either stored in the liver or passed out as waste.

In the 1870s, Dr E von Wolf discovered that the iron content of spinach was 10 times that of any other green vegetable. However, this quickly created a scandal as he had actually misplaced a decimal point in his calculations, meaning that in reality spinach's iron content was about the same as other green vegetables such as broccoli. But, the damage was already done and the character of Popeye was born.

Q. Is brown bread really better than white, and what about wholemeal?

A. White bread is generally thought of by many as worse than brown, but this generally isn't true. Often, brown bread is simply white bread but with colorant added. Similarly, although wholemeal used to be a better option, you no longer get the goodness from all the three parts of the grain as modern, more intensive processing techniques remove many of the B vitamins, as well as minerals such as selenium, found in the grain. For this reason, the best type of bread to eat is wholegrain.

"fat mind, fat body"

Q. What if I can't fit exercise into my day?

A. We can all find a few extra minutes in the day, even if it's just getting up 10 minutes earlier or getting off the bus one stop earlier than normal. This time can be used to exercise; maybe you are cooking a meal and waiting for the pan to boil, you could jog on the spot or hop on an exercise bike in the next room. You could exercise whilst watching TV to make things go faster. Just by finding a few extra minutes, you will be improving your health immeasurably.

Q. Can I drink alcohol?

A. You can drink alcohol, but don't binge. Remember, alcohol contain excess calories that could mean you end up storing more fat. Why not alternate your alcoholic drinks with soft ones.

Q. Can't I have any foods I enjoy?

A. Of course you can, but in moderation. Remember the portion size guidelines and think about how many calories and how much saturated fat is in the food you want. Is there an acceptable replacement that is lower in calories, saturated fat, or has a lower glycemic load, or index? For example, when you want a pizza there is a big difference between a stuffed crust, extra cheese and pepperoni, and a stone-baked, thin crust, non stuffed, lean ham and light mozzarella option. You could further improve the healthiness of the pizza by adding a mixed leaf salad and a sprinkling of olive oil.

Don't be afraid to experiment with your food choices. Often we are afraid of trying new things, but is this fear logical? How do you know you don't like something unless you try it for yourself? Empty your mind of any negative associations you may have built up with the healthier food and replace them with positive ones.

Chapter Three

Remember, the healthier alternative can help you attain your goals and lose those unwanted pounds.

Q. What do I do if I don't have the space to work out at home?

A. You could exercise outside or at the gym, but if you still want to exercise at home, don't worry. Try rearranging your house to make space, not much space is needed for an exercise bike for example. Alternatively you could simply do aerobic exercise in front of your TV to an exercise DVD.

Q. What do I do if I want my partner to lose weight?

A. Being open and honest is important, but don't be confrontational. Tell them it's for their health. Suggest you both need to lose weight and look into activities you could do together, or suggest they take up a hobby they used to enjoy. Remember to be supportive.

Q. What do I do if I don't have time to cook?

A. Generally, home cooked food from fresh ingredients is better for you than prepared food, for a start you actually know exactly what is in it and can tailor the recipe to your needs. However, if you read the back of packets, you can choose healthier options. That said, when I first started cooking for myself, I often felt the same way, but over time I learnt that there are many recipes that take just 20 minutes, for example, stir fries, salads, and grilled food. There are also many recipes that take around 20 minutes to prepare although the cooking time is longer, such as stews, steamed dishes, and roasts. With these meals you can simply put them in the oven, or steamer, set the timer and go do something else. So actually, we all have more time to cook than we think.

Q. Is gluten free food better for me?

A. Gluten free food, a type of protein found in grains like wheat and barley, is designed for people with digestive diseases such as coeliac's disease as their bodies can't tolerate gluten. Gluten free food is no better for you than any other type of food and is often more costly. If you suspect you have a digestive disease like coeliac's, consult your doctor.

Q. Do I have a food allergy or intolerance?

A. A food allergy occurs when someone's own immune system attacks their own body in response to a particular food or ingredient. Food allergies are rare but can be serious, with the most extreme allergies involving nuts and celery. If you suspect you have a food allergy, your doctor can organise tests to eliminate potential causes. A food intolerance is when the body doesn't tolerate a food well, but stops short of a full-blown allergic reaction, an example might be bloating. Many people think they have intolerances when they don't. Common intolerances include dairy (lactose intolerance), and spicy food. If you suspect you have a food intolerance, don't automatically restrict the foods you eat, instead consult a professional, such as your doctor, who can test you.

Q. What are E-numbers?

A. A common misconception is that E-numbers represent artificial additives added to our food. However E-numbers can include potentially helpful, naturally occurring ingredients added to our food. The E in E-numbers just means that the food additive has been passed for safe use in food by the European Union. In general, E numbers from E100 to E199 are colourings, E200 to E299 are preservatives, E300 to E399 are acids, antioxidants, and mineral salts, E400 to E599 are vegetable gums, emulsifiers, stabilisers, and anti-caking agents, E600 and above are flavour enhancers, and E900 to E1500 include all other additives. Some research suggests E-numbers in large quantities may potentially cause harm which has lead to somewhat of a health scare, with the European Union insisting that you are unlikely to consume these additives in a sufficient amount to cause any harm. Other people argue that there is little research looking into the effects of much smaller quantities of these additives when combined together. By preparing foods from fresh ingredients yourself, you can avoid any concerns you have over E-numbers.

Q. What do I do if I fall back into unhealthy habits?

A. In short, don't beat yourself up about it. Relapse is a normal part of the weight loss process, simply remind yourself of all the reasons why you want to cut the weight and restart. Ask yourself why you relapsed and what you can do differently in future? Learn from your mistakes and use this relapse as important feedback, allowing you to be more successful next time. Don't tell yourself, "If I get back to healthy ways I 'may' lose weight," tell yourself you 'will' lose the weight. Each day is part of the learning process and as long as you take on board the messages and lessons that life is teaching you, then you will achieve what your goals.

Q. The people around me are trying to pull me back into bad habits, what can I do?

A. Be strong and remember why you started this journey and all you will achieve by reaching your goals. Many people don't realise they are encouraging bad habits and others may feel alienated by you no longer doing some of the activities you used to do together. Either way, you need to be honest with the people around you and share the way their actions are making you feel in a non confrontational manner. Be calm and be patient. If someone wants you to join in on an unhealthy activity, like going for a takeaway with them, why not suggest an alternative, or if you go, feel good about choosing a healthier option from the menu? That way you can still spend time together without falling into bad habits.

"fat mind, fat body"

Q. Isn't there just a magic weight loss pill I could pop?

A. Whilst it's true that there are weight loss pills on the market, it is also true that the majority of these pills are over hyped and are unlikely to lead to fat loss in the long term. Certain well known brands of diet pill contain a diuretic as the main active ingredient which suggests that most of the weight loss people would experience from using them would be from water loss, and only temporary.

Other pills claim to work by binding the fat or carbohydrate in the food you eat, preventing all of it from being digested. Whilst the theory behind this type of pill is sound, overuse can lead to diarrhoea and problems absorbing fat soluble vitamins. Other products containing L-carnatine, a substance the body uses to transport fat from cells, are also ineffective as the compound is very poorly absorbed by the body and can cause stomach upsets in high amounts. One type of drug you may have heard about is Statins. These do not create weight loss but help reduce cholesterol, and if you have already had a heart attack they can greatly reduce the risk of a second. The problem with Statins is that they don't distinguish between "good" and "bad" cholesterol and there is some evidence this may increase the risk of other diseases such as Parkinson's. Although side-effects from Statins are rare, some of the clinical trials that established these risks excluded participants who in pre-screening showed an immediate reaction and so the risk of side-effects may be greater than that normally stated. The simple truth is that the best way to lose weight is through healthy living and a balanced diet.

Q. Is chocolate really good for me?

A. Most chocolate you see in the shops is high in sugar and saturated fat. Recently there has been some misreporting of a study that showed pure cocoa, one ingredient in the chocolate you eat, to be a powerful antioxidant. The study suggested that one or two small, around 1 cm by 1 cm, cubes of pure chocolate may have a positive health effect, but, as you wouldn't normally be able to buy this type of chocolate, the relevance of this finding is somewhat debatable. Don't believe everything you read in the papers.

Q. Are there any other weight loss tips you could give me?

A. Yes. If you have to have a takeaway, choose a healthier option, chicken breast is often the leanest meat and avoid fatty meats like lamb. If you are having a curry, avoid cream based curries like Kormas and avoid doubling up on your carbohydrate portions by getting naan bread and rice, just choose one or the other. As takeaway portions are often large, you should consider getting one meal between two. Remember though that a healthier alternative to ordering a takeaway is to make something yourself. There are thousands of recipes available online, catering for all levels of cooking skill.

If you are struggling to adapt to a lower sugar diet and you are craving sweet foods, try consuming more sour foods like grapefruit for a couple of days. The taste buds on our tongues are not set in stone and our perception of the sweetness of a food changes. Once your taste buds are adapted to the sour food, sweet foods will seem even more sweet, extremely so, and you will not be able to eat them as comfortably as before, and you may even find that you avoid them altogether.

Another tip is to link foods you like that are bad for you, with foods you dislike. By telling yourself that if you eat the food you desire, you also have to eat something you hate, you are placing a psychological barrier between you and that food. You could also try making yourself exercise before you have a food that is bad for you, say 20, 40, 60 press ups, whatever pushes you beyond your comfort zone.

Finally, as well as creating barriers, try creating positive associations between healthier options (as well as achieving your goals) and the things you enjoy. "If I succeed in losing 1lb next week, I will treat myself to a day at the spa." Try to get your partner, friends, and family involved as they are your support networks. "If I have a low fat lasagne instead of full fat, will you give me a massage tonight?" It is important to know that although this is a personal journey, you are not alone.

Summary

• Your weight loss is personal to you.

• Focus on the language you use relating to weight loss and your health goals, rephrasing things as appropriate.

• Reaffirm your weight loss goals with positive images and associations.

• Calculating the calories you need to burn for weight loss allows you to set attainable goals.

• Calculating the amount of energy burnt off by the exercise you do or want to do also aids in goal setting.

• Replace high glycemic index or load foods with lower glycemic options.

• Replace saturated and trans fats with unsaturated fats instead.

• Reduce your salt intake.

• Get your 5-a-day.

Chapter Three

- Any exercise is better than no exercise and the best activity you can do is one you will do.

- Aim to exercise at a moderate intensity (at least) for two and a half hours a week, split up however you wish.

- Don't believe everything you read in the papers.

- Remember, it takes small steps to cross the pond.

E

½. Pulsating light.
around.
perifery.